Praise for *Inc*

Christine Baxter has written a memoir of enormous proportions – I defy anyone to feel unmoved by this intensely personal and confronting book.

— **John Morrow's** *Pick of the Week*

Dr Christine Baxter has been quietly "rattling the bars" of disability for most of her incredible life. As a young child in England, she suffered from scarlet fever and was placed in confinement away from her family for six months. She just wanted to go home and couldn't understand why she couldn't get through the bars of the hospital door and be with her family. This event had a great impact on not only her life, but the life of Australian children, parents, teachers, governments and institutions – on a global level.

Since the age of 18, a new immigrant to Australia with her family, Dr Baxter has been a pioneer in the way physically and mentally disabled children are cared for and regarded and the quality of support systems for families. In particular, she has rattled the bars of much traditional thought in past decades that such handicapped children are unteachable – forever doomed to an institutionalised life.

This incredibly engaging book is her memoir and is the story of a woman who is modest in blowing her own trumpet, a woman who walks the walk of inclusion for all in society, a woman who has a gift for teaching new ideas.

Dr Baxter's professional accolades are many, including working as a consultant for UNESCO. She tells her story through honest and empathetic eyes, painting the horrors of early treatment of disabled children with a soft brush – an observation, not a judgment. With the help of many passionate and forward-thinking colleagues, Dr Baxter has been able to make a real difference in this field. Her joy is quiet, yet overwhelming.

Although officially retired in 2001, this book is proof that this wonderful woman will continue lobbying for the disabled until her last breath. May there be many more books to come.

— **Wendy O'Hanlon,** *Acres Australia*

This is a great story and I think it would be used extensively in courses where there are students entering the world of disability. It has great pace and leaves readers wanting to go on and see what happens next. I also liked the way the author moved through different time periods of her life and the way she relates them back to her earlier experiences in England. What a wonderful narrative. It is powerful, and congratulations to Dr Baxter on such an engaging and gripping story.

— **Professor Patricia O'Brien**
   Director, Centre for Disability Studies
   The University of Sydney

The subject matter, concerning the inclusion of people with intellectual disability, is very topical in Australia, given ongoing policy developments at both state and commonwealth level, including the recently announced plans for a National Disability Insurance Scheme(NDIS) designed to address many of the issues described in the book. Furthermore, the issue of social inclusion for people with disability is a matter of international concern, as exemplified in the recent proclamation of the United Nations Convention on the Rights of Persons with Disability. This book will make a very valuable contribution to the international literature on this topic.

— **Assoc. Professor Keith McVilly, PhD.**
   School of Psychology, Deakin University

I think it is useful for introductory courses to disability for social work students and for social workers in the disability area and for those in other areas whose work brings them into contact with children who have a disability and their families. I think parents and disability service workers would also be very interested to read it. The memoir gives powerful voice and lends strength to the need for more support for families. My comments on strengths of the manuscript follow:

- Articulation of the relevance of education curricula for children with disability and community inclusion and interesting insight into children's motivation to learn.
- Very effective illustrations of the deprivations of life in institutions and the advantages of alternatives.
- Good to illustrate the disadvantages of services having to rely on donations of money and goods.
- Examples that illustrate how taking action to help children to develop and learn can be an advantage for families as well as the child.
- Articulation of social handicaps, and also of problems with integration.
- Information on the pressures on families, their expressed needs.
- Story of development of the awareness of issues with Maya, the diagnosis, the impact on wider family relationships etc. very honest. Useful for parents dealing with such issues themselves, or those who feel they could have dealt better with them, and for professionals working with families.

— **Dr Meg Gordon, Social Worker**

This is a highly readable story of a rewarding career in disability services. I most strongly recommend it.

— **Dr Josephine Jenkinson, Psychologist and former senior lecturer in the Institute of Special Education and Disability Studies at Deakin University**

This is a very readable life memoir that incorporates a history of special education and the social and political influences on Inclusion over several decades. There are many examples in the book that I could use in my lectures to students about the history of the disability movement towards social inclusion, current challenges, families and services. I see the book as an important resource and university libraries should have copies of it.

— **Dr Janet Owens, Faculty of Health**
  Deakin University, Burwood Campus

This should be read by anybody working in the disability area and also families, as it offers so much hope to them. Medical professionals could also benefit by reading this.

Why is the book needed in the disability sector?

If current international issues concerning inclusion in education and community care are to be resolved, the debate can usefully embrace information from different perspectives. The author's experiences in special education and disability services, and also with a family member who has autism, merge in this very personal memoir. These parallel sources of experience produce a uniquely balanced perspective on disability and inclusion issues.

— **Lynne Maclauchlan**
  Family Carer

'Empty Cradles' (filmed as 'Oranges and Sunshine' and a best-seller in Britain and Australia) is British social worker Margaret Humphrey's story about the lost children of Britain shipped out to Australia. It and 'Inclusion: Battling for Disability' have some features in common, most significantly a determination by their authors to expose dark periods in the history of government services and offer hope for the future. But the children in 'Inclusion' are, on the whole, without a voice to express feelings of distress, disappointment and abandonment. And their parents and carers fear that their call for better services will not be heard and acted upon. Nevertheless, the truth will out in the end, and the events described in this book will contribute to that exposure.

— **RAC**

Unfortunately, and to society's shame, children with mental disabilities right up to the late1970s were kept like cattle in institutions which offered them no stimulus or encouragement to progress to meet their full potential. Parents and carers were given no 'light at the end of the tunnel' and encouraged to place their children in institutions and get on with their 'normal' family lives.

Shunned and locked up, the children were treated little better than caged animals and treated with little respect or humanity. Family members were not encouraged to visit or interact and what a sad and shameful history this has left us with.

Christine Baxter has devoted her life to improving the system which she encountered in the 1960s and 70s. Today, we take for granted that our children will be treated with respect and love; we provide many things to stimulate and encourage growth, both for their minds and their physical wellbeing; and we have a better understanding of the benefit of encouraging anyone with a disability to grow and reach their potential, particularly in taking control of their own lives.

Having said that, there is still a long way to go and with people like Christine Baxter advocating for them, these children, teenagers and adults have a fighting chance to become masters of their own destinies in some cases. For those people with more serious problems, society must learn to be kinder in its understanding of assisting carers and educators into building a better life for them.

Christine Baxter is a woman of compassion and great understanding. It has been a painful journey while reading this book at times. I can only thank God that there are some wonderful and empathetic people out there who are willing to fight for what is right and to pressure governments of the day to provide as much assistance as possible to ensure everyone has a 'fair go'.

— **John Morrow's** *Pick of the Week*

Inclusion

Battling for Disability

Christine Baxter

Published in Australia by Sid Harta Publishers Pty Ltd,
ABN: 46 119 415 842
23 Stirling Crescent, Glen Waverley, Victoria 3150 Australia
Telephone: +61 3 9560 9920, Facsimile: +61 3 9545 1742
E-mail: author@sidharta.com.au

First published in Australia 2012
This edition published 2012
Copyright © Christine Baxter 2012
Cover design, typesetting: Chameleon Print Design

Author photograph: Melbourne Headshot Co

The right of Christine Baxter to be identified as the Author
of the Work has been asserted in accordance with the
Copyright, Designs and Patents Act 1988.

Baxter, Christine
Inclusion: Battling for Disability
ISBN: 1-922086-84-3   EAN13: 978-1-922086-84-6
pp266

viii

About the author

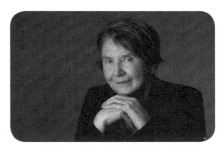

Christine Baxter migrated to Australia from the UK with her parents and three siblings in 1957 and eventually settled in Melbourne, Victoria.

She became a teacher of children with a disability, first teaching at a day training centre in Melbourne and then at a residential special school in Adelaide. In Canberra she was initially employed by the Handicapped Children's Association of the ACT and then, in 1969, following integration in to the education system, became the first teacher-in-charge of the first special pre-school run by the ACT Department of Education and Science.

During the 1970s Chris was employed as a training advisor to day training centres for intellectually disabled children in the state of Victoria. She also taught in the training school run by the Mental Health Authority at St Nicholas Hospital.

When the Institute of Special Education and Disability Studies was established at Burwood in 1976 Chris was seconded as a lecturer and she worked on, through the amalgamation with Deakin University, until 2001. She was invited by UNESCO to be an international consultant in special education and during the 1980s conducted consultancies in Turkey and Burma. She continued her consultancy work with disability services and parent groups over three decades.

Chris gained her PhD in sociology from Monash University in 1986. She was the first researcher in the world to investigate stigma as a stressor for parents and mediators of that stress. In 1988 she won a national research prize awarded by ASID. The monograph series she wrote on *Barriers to Integration* showed how social attitudes, structures, policies and access to support services impact the lives of children and their parents.

When residents from institutions were settled into community housing In the 1980s and '90s Chris was appointed team leader for an evaluation of the Shared Family Care and Permanent Care programs in Victoria. In 1996 she became team leader of the equity access research and development group at Deakin University. She has published many articles on parental stress and social aspects of disability in professional journals, and has co-authored a book on early intervention.

After retiring from the university in 2001, Chris reinvented herself as a writer. *Inclusion* is her first venture into the genre of memoir.

Acknowledgements

I acknowledge with appreciation all of the children, families and colleagues who were involved in the struggle for inclusion that is at the heart of this story. Ethel Temby allowed me to intersperse her memories within the narrative, and I am very grateful to her. Rosemary Crossley and Anne McDonald were also important players in the events I've described. They highlighted the plight of people living in institutions and showed what is possible when residents leave. Many people will be forever grateful for what Ethel, Rosemary and Anne achieved in their very distinctive ways.

(Sadly, Ethel Temby died on the 10th July 2012 aged ninety seven.)

Jan Harper contributed the section on closing down St Nicholas Hospital. I was delighted when she gave me permission to include previously unpublished material in this book. My partner Bob and many friends, colleagues and people in key organisations helped me with feedback at various stages in the project. Several people applied their skills and expertise in a variety of ways, and I am grateful for each and every contribution.

Finally, my nephew Tony, his wife Lyn and their daughter Maya permitted me to intrude into their private lives and to tell this story from my own perspective. They challenged my thinking and revealed the reality of family stress and ways of coping with it and, in an amazingly generous gesture, allowed me to reveal it to a wider audience. We hope that this story throws light on the needs of families like ours.

Note

This personal memoir is set within the historical development of disability services. It is based on my memories aided by conversations, diaries and other documents. To protect the identity of some of the people in the story, family names have often been withheld and many children, officials and people I've been unable to contact have been given a pseudonym. In a few cases their identity has been disguised or merged.

Current disability nomenclature has been used except when specifically indicated otherwise in the text. Much of the dialogue approximates rather than records what was said. The events in this story have been described from my perspective and other participants may well have interpreted them differently.

Some events that happened over time have been merged within a single chapter. Nevertheless, the historical sequence of events is evident as the narrative unfolds.

Readers should note that this is not a documented history of disability services, nor is it a history of the movement towards inclusion. It should be regarded as a small personal anecdotal contribution to the broader historical record and offers one voice among the many others whose perspectives might also add to that history.

Prologue

T he ambulance sped down our street with the horn blaring. The sight of my mother standing at the door with a handkerchief to her eyes told me something terrible must have happened. But lying on a stretcher in the back of that monstrous screaming vehicle I knew only that I was being taken away from home. It would be six long months before I could even touch my mother again.

A very sore throat had confined me to bed and red blotches covered my chest and arms. The doctor looked into my ear. Today, antibiotics would be used to prevent scarlet fever turning into a devastating infection of the ear. But in Britain during the war years, vaccines hadn't been invented. The new wonder drug penicillin was restricted to soldiers fighting the war. In hospital two shadows moved me from the stretcher into a bed in a darkened room. The bed had sides with rails and I woke up thinking I had been locked in a cage. But gone was my strength to rattle the bars.

There was a door to the room with a tiny glass peephole and flashes of shadow meant somebody was there. I must have cried very loudly and a nurse came hurrying in. She explained that the bars were to keep me safe. But I didn't feel safe in this alien place. I just wanted to go home.

After dark my fantasies took form. I saw mice moving across the floor and imagined their cosy home. Each mouse had the name of a family member or friend. Lois had a light grey coat that glowed almost white in the moonlight and she was always

1

happy and smiling, just like my best friend. Irene had large eyes and often sat preening herself, exactly like my older cousin. The very first mouse to scamper back into the shadows after being startled was always Doreen. She had probably run off to feed her pet tortoise on the leaves she'd collected from the lane. Mother was beautifully round and cuddly, and father had dark whiskers. The thin mouse with the dark grey coat, like my grandfather's, could barely be seen behind the rail; probably tending the roses he loved so much.

Every night I joined the mice in their home: mother making tea and me listening to *Children's Hour* on the radio; my friends calling from the door to be let in, and father arriving home with open arms. Fantasy, and life as I'd once known it, merged into one.

When dad was able to take leave from the army, he and my mother came to the hospital on Sunday afternoon at 2; the only visiting time allowed. Parents and children arrived with grandparents, aunts and uncles. They were not allowed to come into the ward, so stood outside in rows three deep, straining to see us through the locked French doors. Inside the ward, the beds were wheeled to form an arc around the doors. Dad was tall, so he politely stood at the rear, craning his neck to see inside and then waving from afar through the small window panes. When it rained we struggled to see any recognisable faces through the bobbing array of umbrellas and rain hats. There were no conversations between us. There were no hugs.

'How can I get to my mother? The question played on my mind for days. The doors from the ward were locked, but there must be another way. By the time Sunday came I'd thought of a plan. An older girl with short blond hair had smiled at me once when we were waiting for our parents to appear. I thought she would be able to release me. It seemed like a good plan. Sunday breakfast was porridge with milk. Then there was stew, with big lumps of potato, for lunch. After our beds had been wheeled into position around the doors I pointed through the bars to the blonde haired girl and asked: 'please can you open it for me?' She shook her head and muttered something about the nurses being angry. 'No, sorry I can't let you out.'

My plan had failed in an instant. Now there was no hope of reaching my family and no way to go home. Mum came and went, 'I want to go home … Please let me go home.' Nobody told my mother her daughter was crying. I put my head back under the covers and waited for the mice to appear.

Our childhood experiences affect later events in ways we don't always understand at the time. So it was in my case.

Chapter 1

Not just a job

By a fortunate set of circumstances I was sitting in the kitchen of my boyfriend's home in Albury, New South Wales, when a whistle announced that the postman had arrived. Max wasn't yet home, so I sat drinking fresh lemonade made by his mother. Mrs. Finch looked pleased when she tore open the envelope and said the letter was from her niece. She clearly wanted to read the letter so, being a kind and hospitable person, she read it out loud. I sat looking out of the window enjoying the cooling drink, but gradually my attention was drawn to the letter. The writer was a teacher of children with disability. And suddenly I was captivated.

Only four months earlier our family had arrived as immigrants to Australia. I was eighteen and believed anything was possible in this new land. I wanted to do something useful in life, 'not just a job'. Perhaps chance events produce answers to personal desires when the search is already in train. And for me the answer came in that letter.

Within a month I'd been accepted into a training course in Melbourne and believed my destiny was sealed.

By the time lectures began I had already visited a day training centre for children with an intellectual disability. From the road I could see children climbing, running and throwing balls in a grassy play area. Inside they were painting at easels and a few were building with blocks on the floor. Sounds of activity were all around and every child was intent on what they were doing. In another room, some of the children said 'hello' or 'what's your name?' I returned home glowing with the conviction that I would soon become a teacher in a centre like this.

This was the era of institutions everywhere in the western world, and Australia was no exception. Several of these large and forbidding places were scattered around Melbourne. Some began at the time of the eugenics movement around 1900 when it was believed that unless 'feeble minded' people were isolated, locked up and kept out of the community they would breed rapidly and increase this 'undesirable' section of society. Females with genes regarded as bad were prevented from having children, first by institutionalisation and later by sterilisation. When the eugenics movement went into decline following Nazi abuses during the Second World War, another reason was found to keep the institutions going. Doctors faced with stressed parents advised them to put their child in an institution.

The person in charge of institutions, as well as everything else run by the Mental Health Authority, was a psychiatrist from Britain by the name of Dr Cunningham Dax. During the first week of our training, he came to welcome this new intake of students. He was a tall, grey-haired man who expected to be noticed when entering a room full of students all eager to hear whatever he wanted to say. When he described the appalling institutional buildings shown to him soon after he took the job, we grimaced with distaste. But he had a plan to dismantle the board and canvas buildings and replace them with better structures. He even described a new brick building that was already under way. It was a timely message of hope for us students.

Children with intellectual disability had only two alternatives through the 1960s and '70s. They might be lucky enough to get into a day training centre like the one I'd seen. Or they could be placed in an institution. In either case, they were excluded from Education Department schools. Instead, as with children in

Britain and the USA, they were classified under a Mental Health Authority.

A shock was in store for us students in the third week of our course. As we stood around the noticeboard trying to decipher the handwritten notes on the timetable, my friend Jenny put her hand to her head and uttered a loud: 'Oh no!'

'This is the week we visit institutions ... and look, it says we'll all be going together in a bus.'

We piled into the bus like schoolchildren going on a picnic, but the jovial mood soon changed. The driver came to a stop outside a grim collection of buildings on the northern outskirts of the city. A nurse came out to meet us. We stood together like a bunch of tourists waiting to be taken on a conducted walking tour. I looked up at the tiny windows, but saw no sign of life.

The nurse opened a huge wooden door with a key and pushed hard with her shoulder to get it to open. Now we were all inside the thick stone walls. The tour had begun.

We walked straight into a ward where about twenty children were sitting on the bare floorboards. It was the only space free of beds. A male ward assistant hovered over the upturned faces while shuffling around on a hard timber chair. 'Sit down' 'sit up'. If a child failed to respond a strong arm pushed or hauled them into position. He wanted to keep these boys sitting together against the wall; nobody was allowed to stand or walk.

I asked the person escorting our group whether the children went to school. Her face left me in no doubt that I'd asked a very stupid question, and then she said:

'No of course not, they are mentally retarded.'

These sad looking children had nowhere to go other than their sleeping quarters. No beaming smiles like those at the day centre. They had nothing at all to do. This was quite clearly a medical facility but we knew that the children couldn't be cured.

We went through another heavy door and into a ward where about twenty empty beds lined the walls. I wondered how the nurses could move between beds that were so close together. Grey and brown linoleum covered the floor. Everything seemed hard, dull and impersonal. My friend Jenny started to shiver. But the temperature hadn't changed.

We went outside into a fenced enclosure. A few young children ran towards us, touching our hands and arms. What did they want to say to us? Our guide told us that they couldn't communicate anything at all. We stood in a bare and featureless yard surrounded by children. There was nothing else for them to do, so I thought novelty might be the reason they were crowding around us with such intensity. But when I turned to go back into the building, two little girls held on to my arms and clung on as though they would never let go. The nurse said sternly: 'pull them away'. I told the children that I had to go back inside and tried to remove their hands from my arms. Still they hung on. The nurse repeated her instruction 'pull them away'. In the end I freed one arm and pulled my other arm from the second child's grasp.

Why did these children hold on so tightly? What did it mean? I stood rigid and strangely conflicted. What should I do? With one determined step I turned my back on those two little girls and walked quickly through the door. But I would never forget their crying faces when I looked back into that desolate yard.

Now we were in a smaller room in a section called administration.

'Please sit on the benches over there.'

A ward assistant pointed to several old wooden benches in front of a white-washed wall. We sat down and soon had writing pads and pens ready.

Jenny whispered: 'Something is going to happen for sure.'

A doctor appeared and gave us a surprisingly cheerful welcome. He was there to help us 'understand the children and the cause of their disability.' Through the door I could see movement in the corridor outside. A very small boy with curly brown hair yelled very loudly and was whisked away back to his ward. An attendant took charge of the waiting children.

One by one, children were brought into the room, while others waited their turn outside. Every child was taken to an area in the centre of the room. From where I was sitting, it looked like the children were being ushered on to a stage. The doctor showed how each of them differed from a 'normal' child. He pointed out differences in head size. A young boy in a wheelchair was required to turn around so that we could more easily see his larger than normal head; 'See the circumference is abnormal for his age'. We looked at the doctor, and tried not to look at the discomforted young boy.

A child with Down syndrome had his head turned by the nurse so that we could see the telltale epicanthic fold on his eye lid. Then the size of his tongue came up for scrutiny. The doctor said to the nurse 'Get him to put out his tongue.' She showed this boy what to do and he obliged. I wondered whether he had a name; was he anything more than a diagnosis of Down syndrome?

Walking problems received special attention, and a young girl dressed only in panties was paraded in front of us students all busily taking notes. Some of the children looked unhappy about being in this parade. Most walked reluctantly past our row of gazing eyes towards an attendant at the other end of the line. The diagnosis and cause of each child's disability was given particular emphasis and spelled out in case any of us got it wrong. Quite abruptly the parade was over and the children returned to their ward.

I was shocked by this pantomime of medical defects in children.

We returned to the bus and sat down without saying a word. On our way back to the training school somebody broke the silence: 'Well thank goodness we are going to see cottages tomorrow.'

The next day, Kew Cottages was on the list to be visited and I looked forward to a more welcoming place in keeping with its name. The institution for children at Kew had recently been officially separated from the Willsmere mental asylum, with its turrets and typical institutional buildings. But on the ground not much had changed. Here was one huge institution for those who, according to the thinking at the time, didn't belong in the community. My image of nice little cottages in the pleasant suburb of Kew was far from the reality of what we saw.

Out on a veranda there were about twenty adults sitting on pots, like oversized versions of those used by toddlers, and open to the weather on a cool day. Twenty visitors stared at them without flinching. No dignity here for anybody. In the day centre there had been a training program. But here, programs for residents were nowhere to be seen.

We walked slowly through one ward, gazing at children who sat around the walls with nothing to do. The children all had basin haircuts that made them look like peas in a pod. Some children were rocking against the wall and banging their heads in the way I learned to recognise as self-stimulation. Was this due to an absence of anything else to do? My mind flashed back to the isolation ward in which I'd been hospitalised for months as a child and a surge of anger and nausea sent me out of the door: 'I want to go home, let me go home' thoughts of my childhood surfaced. I walked around a clump of trees by myself for a while.

Our training officer, Keith Cathcart, was standing at the rear of the group when I returned.

'Are you all right?' he asked.

I nodded. Had he noticed I wasn't coping with this part of our training? I hoped not. My decision to do this course had survived so far. But a difficult meeting with Keith seemed inevitable. I worried that these visits to institutions were our very first test. And I'd just failed the one on stamina.

'Ah! Here is a nice place.'

The nursery building was separate from the rest of the institution. After all those wards, it was a relief to enter a pleasant building on the perimeter of the site. Newly painted walls with some pictures brought smiles to our faces. Sister Eha was in charge of the nursery and as she talked we could see she loved the babies dearly. I later heard that she was responsible for bringing down the death rate in the nursery and making it a comfortable place for the babies to be. But why were they here at all I wondered.

There were about fifteen babies in the nursery on the day we visited and all were under one year old. They were beautiful little babies, but Keith pointed out the early features of Down syndrome. This was the same diagnosis as the children I'd seen clambering over play equipment at the day centre a few weeks earlier. Here at Kew Cottages each baby was wrapped in a blanket; one in every cot. Baby Rowan smiled when I bent over his crib. Some of the babies were awake and their eyes met my own as I talked to them. Sister Eha cradled tiny Bennie in her arms. He turned his face into her uniform and his crying stopped. He was eager for the bottle being prepared just before we left. I took one last look at these babies, not knowing our paths would cross again.

In the late afternoon I boarded the train home and was glad to find a seat by myself where I could think about the events of the day.

I had wanted to take every one of those babies home with me to the room I shared with my sister Pauline. Why were the babies in an institution? What would their future be? Would they ever go to school? Would they someday have interesting things to do? Perhaps they would eventually leave the institution and live at home like everybody else. Hope stirred within.

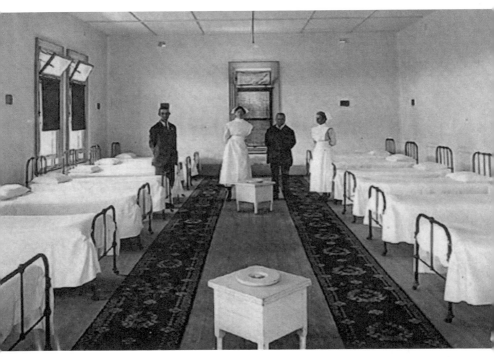

An institution in Australia in the 1940s.
Note the medical focus typical of that time.

Chapter 2

Proud to be a teacher

The nursery at Kew was a disturbing room. Even today, I'm amazed by the stark reminder that in the 1950s and '60s doctors were encouraging parents of children with intellectual disability to place them in an institution. Babies with Down syndrome were easily recognisable at birth and quite a few of those born with this condition that year in Melbourne must have ended up in the nursery at Kew. And we hadn't even seen the umpteen other institutions and babies' homes around Victoria, let alone other states of Australia, Britain and the USA. Advice to parents to place their child in residential care was a very common practise in 1958.

Keith was head of the training school and at the end of the week he asked whether any of us students felt worried by what we had seen. I was the only student to raise a hand. Had everybody else taken all of that horror in their stride? Even my friend Jenny hadn't said a word. On the way out, Keith said: 'Let's have a talk about it.' I liked him a lot, but would he take my admission to be a sign of unsuitability for the course? Perhaps it would be seen as a failure. Horror of horrors! He might even believe that institutions were good places for children with a disability. Perhaps I'd made a mistake about where my future lay.

Keith was a tall, pleasant man with dark greying hair and a craggy face. In class he often asked me what I thought about disability issues and had never once been critical of my answers. But now I was anxious about what he might say. He pointed to a comfortable chair near the window. And we chatted for a while about anything other than what we were there to discuss. He took out his pipe and started to fill it from the tobacco pouch he kept in the top drawer of his desk. He appeared quite relaxed, as though he knew what I would say.

'Tell me what you've been thinking about the visits to institutions this week?'

He spoke in a 'you can tell me anything' kind of way, but he probably hadn't expected such a release of emotion from me. My own childhood experience had added a personal connection to what we had seen. And now this wonderful kindly man wanted to know what I'd been thinking about institutions. My anxiety was dispelled in an instant. Everything came out in a sudden rush of childhood memories.

I told him about being taken away from home in an ambulance. 'I woke up in a bed with rails believing that I'd been locked in a cage.' Keith nodded his head 'The same sort of beds as we saw at Kew.'

'In the isolation ward there was no contact with my family or friends, no toys to play with, no books, and absolutely nothing to do.'

Keith drew on his pipe and nodded. I didn't want to stop:

'When I saw the children in the institution sitting around with nothing to do and unable to go to school … they all looked so very unhappy. It was as though they had been cast out from the world and nobody cared. And when they were paraded in front of us, like they just didn't exist as children …' And so my story ran on.

Keith was a very good listener. He set his pipe aside on his desk and started to talk about the children he knew and the lack of good quality programs in some of the day centres. I listened to stories about parents who had been devastated by the diagnosis of disability and some who were unable to manage their child's behaviour and care. All of this pointed to inadequate services.

'So what needs to be done?' he asked.

He smiled when he heard my answer:

'That's what I need to find out.'

It was past the time for the next lecture and Keith stood up and emptied his pipe.

As I left he said: 'Chris, I think your own experience in hospital will be a driver for what you can now do.'

I wasn't feeling at all confident, but wanted to believe he was right.

Throughout the course I often struggled to come to terms with the field of mental retardation as it was then known. I was nineteen, idealistic and determined to teach in a day training centre. Surely, I thought, if children can attend the centre each day they will not have to go into an institution. And if parents have better support, they will be able to manage their child at home. I was determined to do whatever I could to make it happen. And I was young enough to think that I could.

Pat Kay was in charge of the day centre where I did my practise teaching sessions. She was a tall, slender woman with brown curly hair. I think she was the only registered teacher working in the day centres at that time, so she attracted a lot of respect. Pat was passionate about the arts, and when she introduced drama and music into the program the children enthusiastically joined in. I liked and admired her, and was excited when she invited me to join her teaching staff.

Parents with a child at home had worked hard to establish these day centres for their children. A committee, composed mainly of parents, managed the building and raised funds to supplement government grants for salaries. By the 1960s, graduates of the training course I had just finished were being called teachers, but no political party wanted to increase the budget to provide proper education. So these centres provided the only publicly funded programs for children who were excluded from regular schools.

It was my very first day as a teacher and I walked to the centre from the bus stop feeling more than a little nervous about working with a group of children for a whole day. As I turned into the driveway, a modern building with very large windows came into view. This was the largest centre in Melbourne and Keith had already told me that the committee was the most enterprising in the state. There was a large room for adults who did craft type activities. But the plan was to build a sheltered workshop, where work provided by local factories would mean that the adults could be paid. A kindergarten was being built behind the school building, with features similar to local kindergartens at the time.

I headed for the school. It was the biggest building on the site and faced the car park at one end. A large outdoor play area ran along the length of the building.

Keith had stoked my determination to develop the best education possible for children in this day centre and also to support their parents. I admit to being driven by an ideological zeal to make the institutions redundant by helping to provide a better alternative. The people I'd met during my training believed these children could be trained and occupied, but nobody talked about their education. The confident optimistic side of me wanted to believe they could learn very much more than most people in the day centres expected of them. I guess I'd found a cause to fight for and was determined to find out what these children could do.

High-minded ideas were quickly dispelled by fifteen children noisily tumbling around the floor of our classroom on that first day. Thankfully, a few sat on chairs and waited expectantly to see what would happen. The school building was wonderfully light with a wall of windows overlooking a grassy play area. Every section had modern pull-out cupboards and attractive tables and chairs. The building was divided into junior and senior sections by large folding glass doors. There were two groups in the junior section and my work was with older children from nine to 12 years. Our area was screened off from the next group by three large screens on wheels that could be locked into one another to keep the whole structure intact. Mrs Johns and I had fifteen children each on either side of those screens. By morning tea time a few hyperactive children had already disappeared under the screen into the adjacent group. Just keeping children occupied and happy was enough of an achievement on the first day. When the taxis arrived to take the children home, I breathed a deep sigh of relief.

After a while, children settled into the routine. Running foot-steps and voices heralded their arrival. They opened their bags and put their lunch box in the cupboard and their bag on the hook before going off to the playground until assembly. All the children had an intellectual disability but many also had problems with speech, sight or hearing. Alan had one functional eye and a cleft palate. But he always strode boldly into the classroom. He often put his arms around my legs showing that he was glad to see me before racing into the playground to meet up with his friend Kip, who was always the first to find the newly arranged outdoor equipment. Hugh's family were immigrants from Scotland and had high expectations for their son. He was a very polite boy, but always eager to get out to the playground: 'Good morning Miss – please canna go now?'

Sue preferred to stay indoors, helping me to place the chairs around tables and arrange the flowers in a vase. She had an inoperable hole in her heart but it didn't stop her from helping as much as she could.

In this centre I rarely saw a child who looked sad. There was no disturbing behaviour such as children banging their head against the wall like we had seen in the institution, and the children were soon using the bathroom and dressing without any help.

Every day was a little easier. But the educational program was taking longer to develop than I'd expected. There were routines and timetables but no curriculum in the day centres. I'd been told that a twelve year old with an IQ around 50 would only be capable of doing the same as a preschool aged child in a regular preschool. But I wondered whether their many more years of experience might make quite a lot of difference. In any case I wanted to introduce more challenging activities for these older children than the early childhood ones that my lecturers had liked so much.

First I had to find out what these 'moderately' intellectually disabled children could reasonably be expected to do. So where do you go to get information? I loved the library at Royal Park, so the librarians loved me and went out of their way to search for anything that might be useful. One day Julie, my favourite librarian, said: 'Look at this Chris, it came in today.'

She gave me copy of a program being run at a centre run by a charitable organisation in New Jersey, USA. The program was in paper form, copied on one of the crude printers of the time. It certainly wasn't brilliant by today's standards, but it fired my imagination about what these children might be able to achieve. More paper copies of programs being run at centres in the USA and Britain followed. This material contradicted the thinking of those who believed that these children would not be able to learn. But in Australia, Britain and America, the policy of education departments was firm. These children were uneducable. I hadn't come across anyone in Victoria who was questioning these views. Nobody had said: 'Take another look at what these children can do.'

I was the youngest student ever to have undertaken the course of training and had all the optimism of youth. What's more I didn't like to see children restricted to what departmental officials believed they could do. A teacher, visiting from another centre, said:

'I think you are treading on dangerous ground with your ideas … have you thought about what Keith and the advisors will have to say about what you are doing?'

Yes I would have to explain what I was doing when Keith came on his next visit. But I was determined to find out a few things for myself.

In 1959 we couldn't find a curriculum guide for these children anywhere in Australia, so Pat said that I should write my own. This was exciting. I put the material from the library in a pile and went through each of them to find where there was overlap and agreement. Then, armed with a scale of child development, I observed and tested each child to find out what they could do and listed activities and teaching aids to help them move on to the next step.

My program included speech development, self-help skills and social-community-awareness as well as the already entrenched physical training, music and easel painting. My totally innovative inclusions were community awareness, name and street recognition and number concepts. Nobody believed that these children would be able to read. But I'd seen sign recognition listed on one of the programs from the USA and that was sufficient information for me.

Soon cardboard reproductions of signs used in the newly built Chadstone shopping centre appeared on our display boards, along with traffic lights. We had a lot of fun acting out the meaning of the signs in the classroom, then walking to the shopping centre looking for road signs along the way. The word STOP now had a particularly compelling meaning and not a single child moved when that word was said.

'Curriculum' had not been mentioned on our course. The one I came up with was poor by current standards but in 1959 it was a pretty revolutionary thing to do. Everything we did followed community themes through the year: art, music, number concepts, speech and sight vocabulary were slotted into segments of the general program along with objectives for individual children.

I wanted the children to learn skills they would need to live in the community. Pat had become an encouraging friend and mentor. Other teachers in the centres began to incorporate these subject areas into their programs and the day centre looked increasingly like a school. Sometimes teachers from the other centres criticised us for moving far beyond what was officially approved. But nobody stopped us and when Pat took visitors through the classrooms she talked with pride about what the children were able to do.

Keith came to visit around the middle of the year and walked into my room chuckling:

'What's this I've been hearing about a curriculum?'

I showed him the material that I'd been using and the curricula draft. He didn't say anything about it but his smile was enough.

Before leaving that afternoon he said: 'I would like you to present a paper at the next conference of teachers; will you do it?'

'Of course.'

We laughed together like old friends. Shared understanding emerged in our laughter, but nothing at all was said.

The parents of the children in my group wanted some hope of improvement. Some had been surprised when their child pointed out a sign they recognised while going to the shops. One morning Belinda's mum told me that her daughter counted everything on the dining table while the family were having tea.

'What's the song about a kookaburra and a gum tree?' Mrs Jane asked.

So, standing there in the kitchen, we rehearsed the song that Sue had been attempting to sing.

Oh good next time I'll be able to join in,' her mother said.

And Tim's mother came in smiling one morning eager to tell me about how his new medication was now controlling his seizures.

'He helped to set the table when his grandmother came for lunch last week and, guess what, my mum spoke directly to him for the very first time.'

Tim could now count to five and set a table for that number of family members when his grandmother stayed for a meal. His mother had shown the first sign of being proud of her son and his grandmother was trying to get closer to her grandson now that his seizures were under control. And not one of these parents would have considered residential care.

Despite all the positive signs of hope, one very difficult question troubled many parents:

'Who will look after my child when I'm gone?'

They knew that their child would never grow up to be totally independent and would always require care and support. Equally worrying, was the realisation that they would not always be around to provide that care. What would happen then?

And before long, it happened in the Bray family.

I sometimes talked with Mrs Bray when she was helping in the school kitchen, so I knew that she was caring for her two sons alone. Her boys had bright and sunny dispositions and were popular with all of us teachers. Josh was the eldest. His dark brown hair was always slightly tousled in a fringe and his eyes lit up whenever he thought of something he wanted to say. When help was needed to move a table, he always seemed to be there standing at the other end. But his legs didn't work very well due to muscular dystrophy. Josh sometimes fell to the floor in his eagerness to get to assembly. I once heard him scolding his legs for his disability saying 'come on legs get up.'

Josh's younger brother Kip was in my group. He also loved school and wanted to get the number boards out of the cupboard as soon as he arrived. But when I brought hand puppets to school, along with a bear house and various items of furniture, for speech development, he soon decided that this was his most favourite thing. While preparing the classroom for the afternoon session, a shadow at the window often revealed Kip pushing his nose against the glass in his eagerness to find out 'what's next?' The two brothers always went out to their home-bound taxi together, with Josh carrying his younger brother's bag. Sometimes they linked arms and Kip's shorter thickset body provided a bit of support for Josh's long wobbly legs. I often thought how lucky they were to have one another as well as their very supportive mother.

But as we know, misfortune can change lives very quickly.

One morning, we heard the terrible news that their mother had died at home during an asthma attack. We found out that Josh had run to a neighbour's house saying 'Mummy asleep – not wake up.' Josh's mother couldn't be revived.

Their neighbour faced two distraught boys who had lost their mother. She told us neither boy asked what would happen to them. But they knew what had happened to their mother. And that's why they cried. This neighbour had sometimes allowed them to play in her garden. Now, she tried to comfort them: 'Everything will be all right.'

They really needed a family member or friend to care for them, but would anybody volunteer? Maybe a couple who were unable to have a child would adopt them. Perhaps a family would volunteer to take them into their home. But nobody did.

Josh and Kip were made wards of the state and the authority decided to place them in an institution. We talked gloomily about the terrible future these two little boys would now have. They had been devastated by the death of their mother and now they would lose their friends and everything they enjoyed at the day centre. Would they end up sitting in a ward all day, unable to go to school? It was a painful, upsetting tragedy, but were any of us teachers prepared to take them home? The authority took Josh and Kip away and we never saw them at the centre again.

It was easy for me to say: 'There must be a better way'. But many parents of children at the centre were solely in the care of their mother. And most of these mothers would expect to die before their child. The need for residential care was definitely required in this situation. But the question was, 'What type of care? And who was going to provide it?

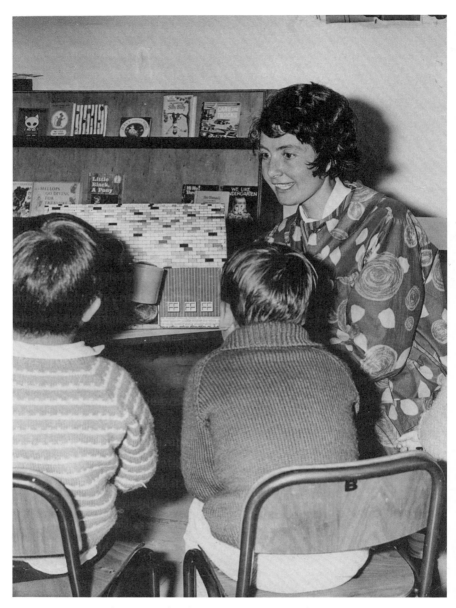

During a language development session at a day training centre
Chris uses a bear puppet to deliver a cup for the children to name.
The children are fully focused on the puppet and not at all on Chris.

Chapter 3

Institutionalised children look over the gate

I was surprised on the first day back at the centre after the term break when Pat Kay told me that she was going to become head teacher at a large residential school for intellectually disabled children in South Australia. An invitation to meet her at a cafe meant that something must be on her mind. The question came as we drank cappuccino: 'Chris, how about moving to Adelaide, to be a teacher in my school?'

My twenty-first birthday had been nearly a year earlier and we had celebrated with tickets to see *My Fair Lady* at the Princess Theatre. By then I'd learned to drive the family car and wanted to be more independent. I suppose the timing was right and leaving the family home was attractive. But first there were some entrenched personal fears to be faced.

Pat had described the residential school as a 'home', but I knew that it was really an institution. The next day I sat on the back deck of our family home with Treasure, our Gordon setter dog, who was stretched out under my chair in the shade. The peace would soon be broken when my brother and sister returned from the riding school they went to every afternoon after school. Worrying thoughts about institutions were on my mind.

I knew that a placement in an institution had been the only solution to the plight of Josh and Kip. Now Pat's invitation caused me to think again about children in residential care. Perhaps here was an opportunity to work with children deprived of a normal family life. Suddenly, Treasure started to bark excitedly as bicycle bells sounded in the driveway.

Next day, Pat told me that the teachers who were being employed by the education department wouldn't be experienced with intellectually disabled children and she needed me to help. She wanted me to work with new teachers joining her staff. Perhaps I just wanted to be needed so it wasn't long before I was packing my bags for Adelaide. The lack of an education department qualification hadn't even crossed my mind.

It was a warm day in Adelaide. Board had been organised with a couple living in a house only a short walk to the beach. Pat had said it was also within easy walking distance of the home. My landlady, Betty, took me to a light and pleasant room. My case contained everything I owned, and that fitted easily into the wardrobe. A wonderful fruity aroma filled the house. When I walked into the kitchen I could see Betty through the window in the garden laying out trays of apricots and peaches on the lawn to be dried. I stared in amazement at the mounds of grapes, with vine leaves attached, on the kitchen table. Then Betty came through the door. She pointed to a dozen jars covering the kitchen table.

'I'm going to pickle the grapes in those jars,' she said. 'You will probably enjoy the pickles and dried fruit.'

'Yes I most certainly will!'

Walking along the beach on that first evening, my overwhelming feeling was one of freedom. The job would be challenging, but it felt good to be living independently at last.

The next morning Pat picked me up for the short drive to the school. The residential and school buildings were spread over several hectares of the beach suburb. Generous people had worked hard to extend it. They wanted it to be a sanctuary and, like institutions elsewhere, this one had grown ever larger. Everything that the children were believed to need had been provided. But it was cut off from the wider community and neighbours living in the surrounding houses probably didn't even know it was there.

The main section was a very large Victorian two storey bluestone building which housed most of the boys in dormitories. Two modern brick additions housed the schoolgirls. There were also several smaller structures used by some older residents who helped around the grounds. After seeing the conditions in institutions in Victoria, this looked like a much better place to me. It was clean and the children were better groomed and dressed.

There were about eighty children in the school, which was run by the education department. And ten of them were in my class. A bunch of noisy children clustered around the door each morning after being walked in line from the home.

Some of the children drew my attention immediately. Brian was taller than the other boys with dark hair, a pleasant face and brown anxious eyes. He wanted to be my helper. During the first week he repeated my every instruction: 'Miss says pack up now.' How does a teacher cope with that? I chose to ignore it but Ann, another child in the group, immediately told him to 'shut up'. Peer pressure worked.

When our routines became better known Brian turned his attention to the classroom, making sure that it was tidy and the chairs were in place. The extraordinary thing about Brian was that he never smiled. Every day there were things that brought a smile to the faces of all the other children, but Brian continued to look glum.

'Try to get a smile from Brian,' became a bit of an obsession for me.

One morning I told the children about finding a possum with a long bushy tail sleeping on the top shelf in the school kitchen.

To add drama to the story I showed them how I had looked at the possum and he had looked at me with wide open eyes. The part of the story the children liked best was when I demonstrated how the possum leapt from the shelf to the bench as the teachers tried to get him out of the door. Then most of the children laughed uproariously. But Brian's lips hardly moved at all. He was a very sad little boy and I wanted to know why.

All the children had been classified as having an intellectual disability, but family breakdown might have been another reason for their being in residential care. And in the case of Brian, as with several other children, I thought that this must have tipped the balance in getting them there.

The star of the classroom was Billie. I first noticed him because of his extraordinarily bright blue eyes. His blonde hair grew out in every direction and he was continually pushing it out of his eyes. He was very observant about everything, including the individual features of the insects that crawled over the windows in summer. I was very worried about Billie because he seemed to be so much more advanced than the other children. So why was he here?

There was no information, but my imagination ranged over some possible reasons. He hadn't spoken about his family, even when encouraged to do so. Perhaps his parents had died and this was the only option available to him. Or maybe his behaviour had not always been as good as it was now and he'd been in trouble with the police. There could have been a breakdown in his family, or perhaps he had failed badly at his previous school. I didn't know why he was here, but as his teacher I had to come up with an appropriate program for him as well as the nine other children in the group. I really didn't know where to start and so we muddled along for a while.

'Billie is very good at art,' said Pat.

I'm not sure how she had made this discovery but it turned out that she was right. We asked him to paint a mural for a forthcoming function.

'Here you are Billie.'

As he took the two paintbrushes I noticed a touch of anxiety as he walked over to a table loaded with bottles of brightly coloured paint. He worked on the floor of the classroom on a very large sheet of treated canvas, placed where he could see his own dormitory building from the window. Within five minutes he'd pencilled an outline of the two storey stone building. Then he mixed and applied the paint while constantly checking through the window to make sure every door and window was in the right place.

After a while Billie stood up laughing about needing to stretch his cramped legs. Soon a relaxed smile showed that he was enjoying the job he'd been given. The green paint jar was almost empty, but it would not be needed again. Billie started to paint children playing on the grass with a ball. I simply watched in amazement. I don't know where he had learned to paint, but most of my colleagues knew that it was not from me. Everybody agreed that the painting was a masterpiece. And the Victorian bluestone building had never looked so good.

Some children had many more learning problems than Billie. Pat Kay had acquired a pet dachshund. She called him Pooch and he sat outside her office every day. But when she moved, he moved, and then children believed to have no speech suddenly found a very good reason to talk. 'Here Pooch' were the first words I heard Michael, a child with Down syndrome from my group, say.

Michael came to life whenever Pooch came over for a pat. It was hard to know what he was saying, but I picked up a few words like 'good dog Pooch' and 'sit here me'. Pooch lay on the floor stretching his long sausage-like body to be patted. Michael loved to run his hand down his black silky coat and to lift up a floppy ear to talk into it. One day I was sure I saw them both poking their tongues and grinning at one another in unison. Boy and dog were oblivious to everything else going on in the room. And as we know, 'happy is a boy with a dog.'

At the beginning of the 1960s the education department of South Australia had not yet produced curricula for children with moderate levels of intellectual disability. This didn't really trouble me. I believed that teaching was all about finding out what children could already do and then taking them on to the next step in their learning. But I was faced with the problem of how to devise a program suited to Michael and his friends as well as the much more advanced Billie, Brian, Tommy and the two girls. It would be impossible to teach the class as a whole. However, if I could make enough teaching aids, the children would be able to work in groups. Most importantly I wanted these children to enjoy school and be eager to learn new things.

One Monday morning I was feeling pretty pleased with the cardboard teaching aids I'd made. But a big problem emerged that struck to the core of what I wanted to do. The children had very little interest in the aids I was so proud of.

'Why do I have to learn about measuring?' and 'I don't want to use the clock.'

There wasn't even a spark of interest in the artificial eggs I'd managed to find for number work and some children didn't even know what the white oval balls were. Billie's red haired friend Tommy had so much potential to learn. But nothing could persuade him that he needed to learn about money. Janet was the prettiest girl in the class and was usually eager to please. This Monday morning, however, she was more interested in yelling at another child, Bobby, who pretended to see insects in her short blonde hair. Neither of them had any interest in the counting aids I had carefully prepared. Some children were not interested in anything.

The problem with overly zealous optimism is that it can so easily turn into despair. After the children left for the day I sat at a table feeling bad. If the children didn't want to learn then there was no point in my teaching.

I had thought the teaching aids I had prepared would grab their interest but they hadn't. I had failed at the most basic task of teaching; to motivate children to learn. I let out a sigh of deep disappointment. Why did these children not want to learn?

Understanding gathered slowly.

The school was on the same block of land as the home and enclosed by a perimeter fence with a gate. And I had never seen any child going out through that gate. Many of the children had been cut off from family life. They had little idea about their neighbourhood or the city of Adelaide, or anything else outside the grounds of the home. After a while it dawned on me what the problem was. These children couldn't connect their school work with their everyday lives on the dormitories. They didn't see the relevance of what they were being asked to do.

Of course! It was their isolation from the community that was the problem. They didn't have a good enough reason to want to learn.

The children didn't even know about some things going on within the home. I found out that they were not allowed to enter the kitchen or laundry or any of the domestic areas. Why would they want to learn about time when none of them had a watch, they rarely saw a clock and went to a meal when the bell rang without associating the bell with the time? Nor did they have a mother or father who could show them why measuring things was important. Money had no relevance to their lives whatsoever; pocket money to spend was unheard of and, in any case, when would they ever be able to visit a shop? There were no books on the wards and the children had no idea about street signs or activities available to children living with their parents at home. With a flash of new understanding I saw children stretching to see over the fence. Yes, they were certainly interested in what was out there.

While walking one lunch time past a building that housed many of the children, I mulled over the problems. How could children living in an institution ever learn about life on the other side of the fence? By then I'd reached the gate and was suddenly struck by the best of all possible thoughts. If the children learned how to use practical community things in school, would they one day know how to use them outside this gate? I was stretching the bow, but it was a target worth trying for.

One day, walking along the main drive I met Michael's older sister. She told me that she visited her brother every Christmas and on his birthday but felt sad about not being allowed to bring a present.

'Why is that?'

'Oh I once brought a book all nicely wrapped up with a card. But an attendant from the home told me that it would cause trouble between the boys.'

This very caring sister had thought it best not to bring her brother a present after that. How would children ever learn to enjoy books if they didn't have any? Would this happen anywhere else other than in a home where large numbers of children were herded together?

Pat came to the rescue by organising for us to use the local library. This meant a weekly walk passing signs, shops and community facilities along the way. The librarian was very good at her job. She was excited by the books in the library and loved having children around who enjoyed them so much. She got to know their interests and found new books to show them every week.

The walk to and from the library was very good for another reason. It meant that the children could take a look at the suburb outside the gate. The children loved seeing the gardens of the houses we passed.

'Look Miss.'

Billie was pointing to a cute garden gate with the number 20. It was just waiting for him to start counting the street numbers by twos; which is exactly what he did as we walked down the road to his chant of 'twenty-two, twenty-four, twenty-six' etc. Brian was more interested in counting the railings that needed a coat of paint. And Janet and Ann held everyone up while working out whether there were more red flowers than yellow ones in a favourite garden. Did neighbours understand that their garden was of interest to children who wanted to learn? Well, time would tell that story.

Children who didn't have space to call their own at home needed to feel that they had it at school. This required a major reorganisation of the classroom.

'Please help me Brian.'

We carried two tables to a corner of the classroom and the serious unsmiling Brian set it up, ever so neatly, with books. Children kept their own borrowed books here with their name on a cardboard bookmark. Three of the children could read a little and went to this area every day. Some were more interested in the pictures.

I knew that the children needed to know much more about what happened in their community. But would they ever be allowed to go out? Help came in an unexpected way. A staff member from the home was very interested in what was happening at school. We quite often talked together about the children.

He understood that they were deprived of many quite ordinary childhood experiences and gained permission to take small groups to the 'footie'. This outing was enjoyable for the game itself, but I ventured: 'Think of all the exciting things the children are going to learn.'

'Do you think Pat will employ me as a teacher?' asked my friend.

'You never know, but then there wouldn't be anybody to help the children learn at the home.'

Permission to go to the footie was an exciting development. The children travelled by train via the local railway station and used the shop at the football ground. They also got to use the railway booking office. Here they would at least learn that money was useful. Only a small number of children were allowed this taste of freedom, but most were from my group. I hoped that it would show them the usefulness of what they were learning at school.

Footie became a passion for the children. And of course they wanted to play that beloved game. They also wanted me to play with them and were rewarded when they yelled 'Kick it to me Miss' or 'You are not allowed to hold on to the ball Miss.'

There was a lot of laughter. But never from Brian; not even a smile. Sometimes at the weekend I called in to see the children play. My colleague from the residential said: 'Better give up your day job – we need you around here.'

Very little progress had been made in special education programs by the education department. Goals and learning objectives for moderately intellectually disabled children were unheard of. So, I came up with my own goal for their education.

The children would learn to understand the community in which the home was located and how things worked in it.

It was a goal that could include every area of curriculum and every aspect of life in the community. The hardest part was working out a program for each and every child. Everything they were learning in the classroom had to be shown to be useful for something they wanted to do outside.

Now there was excitement in our classroom. One of our projects answered the question: How does a railway station work? We collected brochures and information sheets from the local station. That meant we could talk about what we needed for the booking office and to make a signs used at the station and in the carriages. We also made tickets in various categories of price and colour. Brian said: 'Look I've put all the different coloured ones with the prices in bundles.'

Meantime Tommy was placing coins from the cash box next to the ticket price. Billie was running the cash box, writing down the amount each morning and counting it out on returning it to me. At the end of the counting he would say: 'All the money is correct.' And, after a while it was, because Billie was learning faster than any of his friends.

We picked up a railway map with the stations listed. Some children copied the names on to lists with the price of tickets written in columns. Billie took on the role of booking officer and helped a few of the less able children to place coins according to the correct price of the ticket. Soon Billie was able to add up any combination of coins without any difficulty. Janet and Ann were also very interested in money and their skills were developing surprisingly quickly.

Using a Next Train sign and a clock face, we connected the stations on that line to the times listed. Children who had previously looked bored and disinterested started to concentrate intently on what they were doing. They moved around with a purpose. There was conversation in groups. Some were overly passionate about what they were doing and squabbled a bit. So I gave the children individual roles to perform and the squabbling settled down.

A project about Adelaide and surrounding areas led to an incident involving Billie. I'd picked up copies of a map of South Australia from the local tourist centre. In the same bundle were photos of regional towns and suburbs. Several children were able to match the name on the photo and the name on the map. The more advanced children worked on separate projects with different destinations. They recorded the order of towns along the road or the rail link to the destination. Two children were able to select their own destination town and Billie pleaded: 'Can I have Whyalla?'

I was pleased that Billie knew the name of a town quite a long way from Adelaide. He was totally absorbed in this task; continually checking with me that he had got the order of place names along the route right.

It should have set the alarm bell ringing, but it didn't.

On the Monday morning of the following week I was worried when Pat told me that Billie had left the home on Saturday morning without telling anyone. It was a surprise because I really believed that he was enjoying school. Why would he want to miss even a day of it? Fortunately he was brought back later that same morning.

'I wanted you here in the map reading group this morning Billie,' I told him

He pushed a strand of hair out of his eye and said: 'But I was going to come back on Monday for school Miss Baxter.'

'So what stopped you?'

'A policeman came and stopped me.'

'Were you lost?'

'No I had my map.'

Billie put his hand in his pocket and took out a much folded copy of the map of South Australia he'd been working on the previous week. Later, I was told that the police had been called by a car driver when Billie was trying to hitch his third ride of the day. And yes, he was on his way to his destination town of Whyalla. I was silently amazed by his map reading cleverness.

As Billie left the classroom at the end of the day, he said,

'I'm going to be a policeman Miss Baxter – they know every road in South Australia.'

'So you'll need to stay around here and do some more map reading then?'

He nodded.

At the door he turned his head and said 'Sorry Miss Baxter.'

Billie had been classified as intellectually disabled but he understood that disappointment was the reason for my grumpy welcome home.

I walked to the gate feeling thoughtful and sad. Why was such a capable boy in this place? I hoped that Billie would eventually be free to live and travel by himself and get a job that he liked. The incident stoked my resolve always to hope that he and his classmates would one day do just that.

By then, however, our walks to the library had revealed that life outside the institution was not going to be easy for any of these children. Walking with the children down neighbourhood streets was usually a pleasure. But one day a bunch of boys from the primary school were standing together on the other side of the road. One of them called out:

'Retard! Retard! Retard!'

The taunt landed like a bolt of lightning on the leaders of our group. Nobody moved. Brian scowled fiercely in the direction of the boys in school uniforms, Ann looked ready to burst into tears. I walked to the front of the group and, with a strong gesture with my hand, pointed in the direction the boys over the road should go. They went, and our group walked on. Michael was having trouble holding on to my hand and Billie was in his usual place by my side. After a while he said,

'That's what they called me at school.'

'But it's not what they call you at this school Billie so you should just ignore things like that.'

Tommy's red hair was bright in the sunlight and he said with feeling,

'They are just silly little boys.'

None of us disagreed with that. But then a remarkable thing happened. I turned around and my eyes met Brian's. It wasn't a huge smile, just a nice upward movement of his lips. Why would he smile at a comment from Tommy like that? Did Brian harbour hurtful taunts from his earlier life? Perhaps it was Tommy's dismissal of the taunt that appealed to him. Perhaps it was the strong feeling that Tommy had expressed. In any case Brian had shown that he could smile. It was a breakthrough.

The reaction of neighbours varied between the extremes of effusive sympathy to outright fear, anger and antagonism. On one occasion a neighbour complained about our relaxed snake formation as we walked to the library. I was shocked when she said:

'My home might be robbed and what about little Vinnie next door? He could be attacked when he plays on his bike in the garden.'

Indignation welled up in defence of my wonderful children. I knew they could do no wrong.

'This is the best group of children you could ever know – they would do no such thing.'

I said it with absolute conviction, but the words were too passionately expressed. This neighbour had no means of knowing these children and I shouldn't have given her that indignant response. Billie's smile had a touch of embarrassment. We all settled down and walked back to the school in silence.

Our return coincided with a big announcement. The word was out that the school inspector was coming the following week.

The news put the teachers into a state of nervous hyperactivity. I had no idea what to expect and was concerned about whether the inspector would understand what we were trying to achieve.

The following Monday a tall man with greying hair strode down the path outside our window. Ours was a demonstration classroom and we were used to having visitors, so everyone just got on with their work when the inspector arrived. Janet was always the first to attract attention and asked the inspector:

'Would you like to sit with me?'

He nodded and spoke with enthusiasm:

'It's very nice to be asked.'

The inspector was relaxed and enjoying the friendly reception. Everything went well after that. He sat in our classroom talking to children about their books and their projects, watching an activity session and then talking with me in the lunch break. He understood that these children required a different classroom arrangement and liked the 'innovative approach' we were taking. But, then, at that time any attempt to have an appropriate education program and curriculum would have been classified as innovative. When the assessment arrived in the post, he had been very generous in his rating.

As my third year of teaching in Adelaide drew to a close, I found myself becoming increasingly reflective. Despite stumbling beginnings, I knew that the children had benefited greatly from being in this education department school. But for me there were a few personal issues to resolve.

My children had returned to their dormitory on the last day of term. I was restless and decided to walk on the beach for a while. A group of boys from the local primary school were building castles and connecting moats in the sand. Churning water was moving further and further up the sand. I sat on a mound staring into the distance and watching the encroaching tide.

Thoughts about the future came in a rush:

'All children, including those in the day training centres in Victoria and everywhere else, should have access to education department schools like these boys.'

And yes, 'every child should have the right to go to school.'

The inevitability of what would happen when the next wave reached the castle was there for all to see.

I knew that teachers working in special education in the future would need a basic education qualification as well as one in special education. A boy in yellow shorts yelled,

'A wave's coming in.'

Thoughts churned in my mind,

'I only have a specialist qualification.'

The first sandcastle disintegrated into the tide. Yes it was inevitable.

My qualifications had been accepted by the education department and I had completed the core unit of training it had required. But I knew the teachers of the future would need a longer course of training for this job. I started to feel quite vulnerable. The children jumped around in excitement as the tiny moats were swamped and the last castle fell into the surrounding sand. I left quickly, knowing that my bags had to be packed for the summer term break in Melbourne.

Before leaving Adelaide the next day, I walked past the buildings that housed most of the children in my group. Nobody was around. Why was I here? There was no reason at all. I started to wonder what would happen in the future. Would the children ever leave this place and get jobs outside? Would they ever be able to live normal lives in the community? And if I left now, would I find out what happened to them in the future? Yes, of course, Pat would keep me informed.

I reached the road, in sight of the oval where some of my children were playing footie.

'Bye,' yelled Billie and all the other children waved.

My bag fell to the ground and I waved both arms at the same time. I could never forget these children. It felt like they were embedded in my life. A distant voice said: 'Never become too emotionally attached to the children you teach.' I remembered Keith's word of warning. But now it was too late. I travelled to Melbourne for the summer holiday, knowing that something had to be done.

Chapter 4

Hard way to get an education

T eaching in Adelaide had opened my eyes to some personally challenging realities. First was the realisation that children of all abilities should have access to an education department school with well-trained teachers. This carried a sharp reminder that my own schooling was inadequate for the job I wanted to do. Education was not only a problem for the children I taught, it was also a problem for me. Churning emotions plunged me back into childhood memories.

Following my hospitalisation and home-bound convalescence as a six year old, school was a bad experience for me. In some ways my schooling was a comedy of post-war errors although there had been little to smile about at the time. I was a difficult child to educate. Not only had the hearing in one of my ears been destroyed by infection, but I'd missed a whole year of schooling. The shortage of skilled teachers after the war, along with my own inclination to withdraw whenever a problem arose, further hampered my progress.

On returning to school after a whole year away, I was promoted with my age grade as though nothing had happened. I looked at the blackboard without understanding any of the tasks we'd been asked to do. But that long stay in hospital had taught me how to withdraw to a safe space in my own mind. The teacher described me as 'a quiet child' to my mother. Fortunately it was my mother who recognised my misery.

Every day mum arrived at the school gates with a small bottle of warmed orange juice prepared from a government issued concentrate. At recess time she passed the bottle through the railings to me with a few sultanas. Mum helped me to survive the return to school emotionally, but nobody could stem my educational decline.

The school was of good architectural design with classrooms arranged around a quadrangle and a modern hall at one end. I went through these primary years in an uncomprehending fog. Perhaps my teachers believed that a child should be able to catch up, but I never did. There was no assessment of my level of learning, no remedial education and I was punished by my teacher for not doing the work correctly:

'The 2 goes under the 30 not at the side, you can't add the figures that way you silly girl.'

Arithmetic was my biggest problem. Having missed several lessons in first class and almost all of those in second, even the organisation of figures on the page was a total mystery to me. I looked at the page without understanding a single thing. So how do you teach a failing child? My teacher's solution was to punish,

'Sit here, perhaps it will make you do better.'

She pointed to the table next to her desk, where my classmates could stare at my embarrassment.

'This is the place for a dunce in arithmetic.'

That was where I sat all day. Who was going to teach me how to these sums? No teaching, only humiliation. And for me failure continued.

Using books from Sunday school and a tattered copy of *Wind in the Willows* my father helped me to read. Never was I taught at school what I'd missed while in hospital. Even my hearing problem was unrecognised.

Quiet children like me were placed in the very back row of the classroom, in the worst possible position for a child without any functional hearing in one ear. I'm confident that such a thing couldn't happen today because regulations would require better co-ordination between the hospital specialist and the school. My failure in arithmetic and writing persisted throughout primary school.

Examination fever arrived. In the months leading up to the eleven plus examination used throughout England to stream children for secondary schooling, there was a lot of tension at school. The examination had been touted as a means of streaming children into the secondary school best suited to their ability level and job prospects. There was plenty of public criticism of the examination. It was viewed by many people as being unfair, with some arguing that poverty and unequal rates of child development meant that this form of streaming reduced educational opportunities for children.

There was a buzz of pre-examination chatter as we gloomily ate our government subsidised lunches and made patterns with spilled sago pudding along the tables in the school canteen. Some of us were uncomfortably aware that this test could determine our future lives. Several of my classmates wanted to be typists or shop assistants. Others talked about working in a factory, and one thought the factory down the road would be the most likely option for her. A girl from Wales boldly revealed that she wanted to run her own hat shop in Cardiff.

'I want to be a teacher,' my friend Kerry said.

We stared at her in disbelief.

'I mean a good teacher,' she said.

As the two of us intentionally slurped our milk through bent straws, I whispered my own equally uppity dream:

'I want to be a physical therapist like the one I liked in the hospital.' Then, more loudly, 'I hope I will never have to work in the mill.'

Along with my school friends, I sometimes had to deliver a message to my mother in the cotton mill where she worked every day. The loud clack-clack of the looms prevented ordinary conversation, but the weavers found a way. They communicated using a combination of sign language and exaggerated mouthing of words without a single sound being uttered. First they would make eye contact and then point in the direction of the person or object being communicated about; silently forming the words in long conversations. I sometimes sat on a stool, fascinated by this very different way of making oneself understood. The noise of the clattering looms was unbearable, however, and we left as soon as we could.

I prayed every night that I wouldn't have to work in the mill.

The public debate about the big examination went on. All the children in my class had been disadvantaged by poverty, poor schooling and post war chaos. Yet we all had our dreams for the future. We knew that failing this examination would be a barrier to what we might otherwise be able to do.

Two weeks before the examination my father brought home a set of books from a bookseller who promised that they would help me pass the exam. I sat with dad at the kitchen table doing the exercises. He read out the questions to me one by one and then checked the answer sheet to find out whether I'd got it right. Dad claimed that he learned a lot from these books. I made no such claim and many of my answers were wrong.

The day of the examination arrived.

'What's this?'

I felt a furry object that turned out to be a rabbit tail being pushed into my pocket by my mother.

'It's to bring you luck.'

I needed a lot more than luck. It was no surprise to anyone when I failed the examination. When I met up with my friend

Kerry at school after the results came out, she looked very unhappy.

'Now I don't know what I can do'

We sat on a wall in the playground and glumly drank the government provided milk. I walked home feeling that this had been a particularly bad day at school. My grandfather offered a consoling story about how Winston Churchill had done badly at school but I recognised his name as being the old man with a cigar in the newsreels and didn't want to imitate his success.

School never got very much better for me. Informal learning was another matter. It reached a high point during school holidays with my aunt and uncle. They opened up new experiences in reading. At home we had only a few books. The bible was always kept on the hallway cabinet, ready to be picked up on our way to church. We also had many volumes of Charles Dickens and a paperback edition of *Sex in Marriage* that was kept out of view at the back of a cupboard and which I secretly opened when mum was out shopping. There were a few pamphlets and paper-backed books on moral issues brought home by dad from church conventions. But it was the school holidays that taught me it was possible to read for pleasure.

Every summer holiday I was taken by my uncle to the Lewis store in central Manchester to select a book. He leaned against a convenient wall, waiting patiently while I went through every shelf, eventually choosing a book because of the picture on the cover. The most valued holidays were those at the home of my aunt's friend in Bowdon. He was a medical doctor and his wife a wonderfully generous and hospitable woman. Their children, Margaret and Vi, were of a similar age to me and we sometimes rode our bikes around Bowdon and through Dunham Park. During school holidays my aunt and uncle looked after their beautiful house.

The house was three storeys high and had a white-washed cellar with a green table tennis table and a tub full of eggs in preserving fluid. The highlight for me was the books in each of the bedrooms. When Vi saw me looking intently at the rows of brightly coloured books on shelves that went up to the ceiling, she said:

'You can read them all if you like.'

This was a turning point for me. Books transported me to new places and new experiences and I became totally immersed in the lives of the fictional characters. I read every book written by Enid Blyton and finished several by torchlight under the bedcovers after dark. Reading to find out how things work in the world was just as much fun.

My favourite spot for reading was in a gaily striped deck-chair with a yellow canopy, set up on the small grassy terrace at the back of the house. The aroma of raspberries growing in a nearby plot wafted around me in the late afternoon. For days on end, through sun and showers, I sat on that deck-chair with my fictional friends. I'd learned that reading could be one of the most enjoyable experiences in life.

Back at school we'd been streamed for low level jobs and that's how it would turn out to be. I was determined not to work in that horrible cotton mill like my mother. So what could I do? What could I be? Dad decided that he would run his own business from the front room of our house and I could work for him by using an electric router on the wallpaper print rollers.

There was never any doubt that I would leave school at the age of fifteen. I looked forward to it, although working for father was not what I had in mind. A teacher at my school intervened in dad's plan. She sent me for an interview at Leaders dress shop in central Blackburn during a lunch break.

As a junior assistant, I was paid to make tea for the very

sophisticated saleswomen. One of the tasks was to pick up pins that had accidentally dropped to the floor during alterations. Up and down and into every cubicle I went, trying to attract pins with a red magnet on the end of a piece of string. Then, in order to find any pins lurking under chairs and cabinets, I crawled along the plush red carpet throwing the magnet under cupboards and retrieving the pins. The rest of the day was spent in the packing room with lengths of tissue and cardboard boxes.

My future looked very bleak at the age of fifteen.

Then an opportunity for emigration came and by the time I was eighteen our family was heading for Australia. That changed everything.

As the ship came into a berth at Port Melbourne I felt that anything was possible in this new land. And that's how it turned out to be. One thing led to another and my acceptance into the course of training in Melbourne was based on only six months of experience as a kindergarten assistant. Nobody had even asked about my years of schooling. If they had, perhaps they would have been surprised to know that I'd left school one week before I turned fifteen.

Now in Adelaide, having completed the only additional unit the education department required of me, I was confronted with a new reality. My job was secure for the time being, but what would the future hold? I knew that the children deserved very well trained teachers. So increasing my own education was essential. The burning question was: 'How can I get an education at the age of twenty five?'

While staying with the family in Melbourne during the term break, an opportunity came. An advertisement in the newspaper said that a consultant would be at the University of Melbourne to interview adults about continuing their education. Could this be the solution?

I picked up the phone and rang the number straight away. My bold question to the consultant was: 'What do I need to do to qualify for entry to university?' He referred me to Taylors College to study for the matriculation examination awarded by the university and gave me the required forms.

Things happened quickly. Within the week I'd been accepted as a mature age student. By then I had a little money in my account and knew that it would be sufficient to cover a year without a salary. After that, well ...

My fellow students were years younger than me, but that didn't seem to be a problem. We all needed to study hard. And we all had to wear a uniform; even me at the age of twenty five. A highlight of that year was studying in the state library in Swanston Street in the iconic reading room with its beautiful domed skylight and ornate work-tables with their impressive green lamps.

After the results came out I felt excited and energised by feelings of success. Taking the long track around the lake near our family home in Nunawading, I found myself walking unusually quickly. It had taken a long time, but it felt like I'd faced my demons and won. And, in egalitarian Australia, anything was possible.

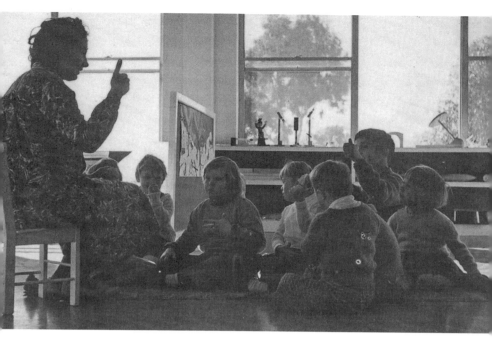

In the 1960s these children were regarded as uneducable and were barred
from attending education department schools and preschools.
The pictures show that they were able to learn if given the opportunity.

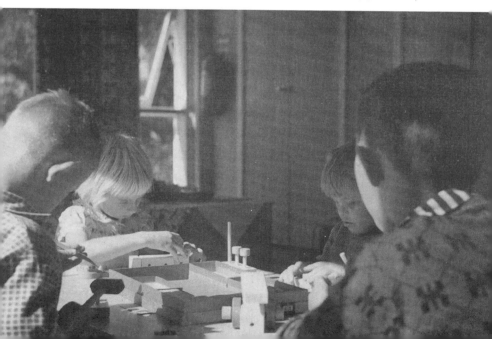

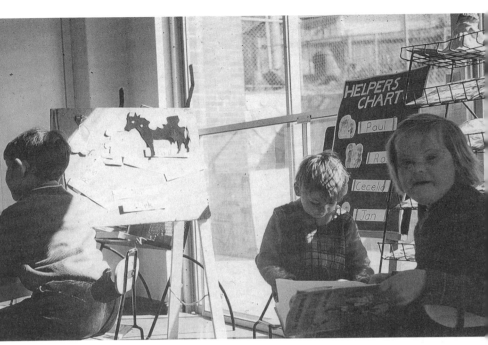

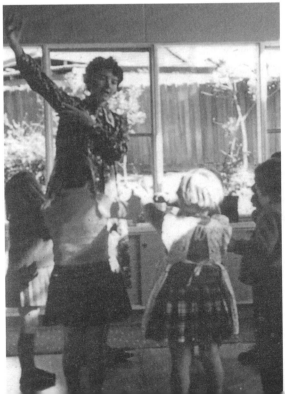

Chapter 5

A model city

After a year out of the workforce, I needed to earn some money quickly. Quite out of the blue a letter arrived with an invitation to visit a day centre for intellectually disabled children in Canberra. It turned out that the secretary of the centre had met Pat Kay at a conference and asked whether she knew anybody suitable to head their preschool and training centre.

Standing at the railway station with all my worldly wealth in my purse, I managed to pay for a rail ticket on the overnight sleeper train to Yass and a connecting bus to Canberra. The bus was already waiting as the train drew into Yass station early in the morning. The driver, a cheerful middle-aged local man, excitedly pointed to his home as he drove past it and invited us all to wave to a wife who couldn't be seen.

Now the bus was on the narrow winding road to Canberra. The driver stopped several times to deliver newspapers and provisions to houses and shops along the way. I sat in the middle of the bus, staring out of the window at men and women sleepily emerging from cottages to collect their goods. A woman in a pink cotton dressing gown held on to a sleepy child in one arm and picked up a package with the other. Older children, dressed ready for school, waved as the bus moved on. I leaned back into the comfort of my seat. Then suddenly, out of rural Australia and cradled between three mountain peaks, arose the national capital of Australia, the sun was already shining on its tallest buildings, although in 1965 it was a very much smaller place than it is now.

The expected job interview never happened. The secretary of the association had organised for parents to bring their children to the temporary building that served as a play centre. And I was to be their teacher for the day. It felt great to be with children and their parents again. By the afternoon, a friendly conversation contained an invitation to become the first paid teacher-in-charge of the Koomarri Pre-School and Training Centre. I headed back to Melbourne by sleeper train the same night.

My bunk on the train was surprisingly comfortable but it was difficult to sleep on the speeding train. I lay thinking about the events of the day. Did I really want to go to Canberra? Mainly positive thoughts sprang to mind. Having overall responsibility for the centre would give me the freedom to work for what I valued. Contact with parents would be expected and I was keen to try out some new ideas. I knew that the centre wasn't integrated within the Department of Education, but felt optimistic that this would happen in the enlightened city of Canberra. It was something important to work towards.

I was a little worried about 'all that responsibility' but by the time the train came in to Spencer Street station I'd convinced myself I would cope. Somehow, my time in Adelaide and the year spent improving my education in Melbourne had boosted my confidence. I heard my mother's distant voice saying 'Pride goes before a fall,' but ignored that warning.

This was an era in which charitable organisations were pioneering disability services. On a hot day at the end of January 1965, I arrived in Canberra to begin my new job. The taxi drew alongside a large rather angular red brick building that stood out against the native dryandra forest covering the slopes of Black Mountain.

The secretary welcomed me inside. She was a slightly built woman with a speedy brain, a caring attitude and was never short of something to say. It felt like a meeting between friends. When she introduced me to the supervisor of the sheltered workshop we instantly knew that we would all get on. But where were the children? It turned out that we had to prepare the new building before they arrived.

The preschool and training centre was on the ground floor of the building and the sheltered workshop on the upper floor. I was sitting at a table surrounded by boxes when the development officer appeared at the bottom of the stairs. He was smallish rotund man with steel grey hair, a voice of authority and a hand with the power to move anything it encountered. He quickly swept two of my boxes to the far end of the table and spread a roll of paper in front of us: 'I want you to take a look at these drawings.'

I was eager to know what this man thought about the future of the centre and to find out whether integration with the Department of Education was in his mind. Perhaps this was a good opportunity. Instead, he wanted me to look at drawings of the completed building in which we sat.

We studied the drawings for a while and discussed every feature of the building. He pointed out its great flexibility and how it could be adapted for any purpose the association might choose. That was a great start. It meant that the building could be used for other purposes no matter what happened to the kindergarten. I said: 'So the space will be useful, even if the kindergarten is taken over by the Department of Education?'

The development officer looked surprised by my question and I wondered whether I'd been too bold. His answer stunned me.

'There is nothing about a kindergarten on the plan drawn up by our planning commission.'

This planning commission was obviously very important, so I asked:

'What was this planning authority set up to do?'

His answer was one most residents of Canberra knew very well but was not what I wanted to hear:

'Nothing happens in this city without the approval of the National Capital Development Commission.'

My desire to get the preschool integrated into the education department had hit its first obstacle.

The children arrived in eight taxis each morning. I'd set up two groups of kindergarten children. The third group was for older children who had been declared 'not suitable' for entry because of a more severe level of disability than was acceptable at the special school. But there was plenty they could learn.

Two of the children in the kindergarten had autism. Sandy often came to the centre without a skerrick of clothing on her body. The taxi driver gave me a rueful smile while handing over a bundle of clothes that she had spent the entire journey from home removing. Once inside, she ran gleefully from one end of the building to the other and then climbed up on to a table to sit on the teaching aids that I'd carefully set ready for the day. Only then, did she look directly at me. I was relieved when Mrs Grant and Mrs Viller were employed as assistant teachers. This meant that we would be able to set up three groups.

With the goal of integration into the education department in mind, I ran a program for the kindergarten aged children much like those in regular preschools. Visitors from the diplomatic embassies and service clubs were often surprised by what the children could do. It pleased me when a visitor said 'it's just like my local kindergarten' because that's exactly what I wanted it to be.

A highlight of the day was when children sat on a mat in the largest of the rooms. Every child took their turn to take something from a box on the table and name what had been selected. Action songs using arms and hands, with fingers pointing at nose, eyes, mouth or ear, were very popular. Yes, it was a kindergarten!

Living in the national capital was exciting. Years earlier we had visited Canberra briefly as newly arrived immigrants. At that time we saw cattle grazing where the lake was destined to be. When I moved to Canberra in 1965, the Burley Griffin Plan was being implemented and the city was taking shape as the national capital. Australians tend to either hate Canberra or love it and I was in the latter group. Civic was the centre of life in the city. New suburbs were under way and would soon become homes for the many young families relocating to the capital. And of course some of those families would include a child with a disability.

In many ways Canberra was a model city for young families and children so long as none of them had a disability. Very few children had grandparents living in Canberra, or any other family member able to help. A government funded crèche was there for parents who wanted to shop for a while in Civic or attend appointments without their child. They could drop off their child for an hour or two for a very small fee. Preschool centres had been set up in the older suburbs and new ones were already going up in those still being developed.

Despite the impressive range in children's services, there wasn't a single government provided facility for young children with an intellectual disability. And these children were well and truly excluded from services used by everybody else. A brochure I picked up from an information stand proclaimed that the preschool office was in the Department of Education and Science and was responsible for all kindergartens. But 'all' didn't include children with a disability. Our kindergarten was not listed, and from my perspective it looked like our children didn't belong.

All of us teachers were grateful to the organisation running the centre and glad of the volunteers from the embassies and service organisations in Canberra. But equal access to education for the children was my aim. The planning commission problem was now firmly in my mind. In fact it was often the development officer who raised these planning issues with me.

One day I stood with him admiring the building, saying: 'How fortunate that it is such an adaptable space.' It had been a relief to know that the space could be used for any of the services run by the association. In fact a much needed expansion of the sheltered workshop was already being discussed.

As we talked, the development officer dropped another bombshell. Apparently, there was a 'five year publicity plan'. Our children certainly looked cute in the brochures, but five years! My inner voice said 'Good heavens, I hope not. Surely these children have a right to the early childhood education services that other children in Canberra have had for a long time.'

Hope for the kindergarten seemed to be slipping away. In addition to the planning commission, it looked as if the development officer would be a further obstacle to integration. This conversation made me anxious. I knew that I would have to tread carefully in the first year. But after that I was determined to push for the rights of children who had been excluded from 'the plan' for this model city. In the meantime there was a long list of parents I wanted to visit.

For the first time, my work with children at the centre also brought a lot of contact with families. They would be able to share information about their child with me and I could try to answer any questions they wanted to raise. There was a category called 'Father's Occupation' on the application form used by the association. It seems rather quaint today. The fathers of children at the centre represented every category of the Canberra population: many were in the public service, a doctor at the Canberra hospital, several tradesmen fathers were working on the new suburbs, six were in small businesses, one was a CSIRO scientist and one was a lawyer. I wanted to visit as many of them as possible.

The secretary got permission for me to travel with children returning home at lunch time in their shared cab. I hoped that we could work together on programs. It was on these visits that I began to understand what some families were going through at home.

One sunny winter Tuesday, I went to see a mother about a child who was listed as having Down syndrome but wasn't attending our kindergarten. The taxi drew into the driveway of a modest house surrounded by several others in much the same style. A letter had explained that a visit would be made on Tuesday at 12.15pm, but there was no response to the bell. A neighbour put her head over the side fence and said that Mrs May was at work but I would be able to see her child through the front window. Sure enough, when I turned to the window at the side of the door, there was a small fair-haired boy with Down syndrome lying flat on his back in a cot.

It was lunch time and Mrs May strode quickly down the path as I was about to leave.

'Sorry I got delayed at work.'

We sat on the only two chairs in the room. When she lifted her child Jack on to her knee he didn't seem able to sit without the support of his mother's arm. The file at the centre showed that he was six years old, but his movements were like that of a baby and he was very small for his age. My mind went back to my own childhood experience of losing the ability to walk after lying in a hospital bed for so long. Here was a child who couldn't seem to sit by himself, let alone walk.

Mrs May slowly relaxed as we chatted about the preschool for children like Jack. Then, in emotional bursts of broken English, her story came out. She had been in the migrant hostel at Bonegilla when her son was born. Not long after Jack's disability was diagnosed her husband had left them and returned to his homeland, leaving no address.

As we talked, Mrs May took a spoon from a kitchen drawer and a container of baby mash from the cupboard and started to feed her son. She wept freely while describing how her husband had left her to manage alone. She knew that it would be necessary to get a job as well as caring for her handicapped baby. Now, nearly five years later, this tearful mother sat in front of me feeding her son like the baby he had always been. My concern for Jack now firmly encompassed his mother.

Jack's mother had no expectation that her son would ever be able to walk, or even sit or stand. Even the three year old children with Down syndrome in our kindergarten were doing very much more than six year old Jack. Mrs May didn't have family members living in Australia and hadn't heard of a service that could help. So each weekday morning she left her son in his cot before going to work.

I watched Jack being returned to the cot for his lonely afternoon, sickened by the thought that a child living at home could be as confined and isolated as those in institutions. What could we do to help this family? It was so very depressing. Jack needed what our centre offered and his mother needed to work.

'Are we to have another child joining our group?'

Mrs Grant was eager to find out what had happened on the home visit I had made earlier in the day. She was outraged when I told her the story and believed the child protection authorities should be called.

'But would that help Jack or his mother?'

It was just as important to find a solution to Mrs May's problem as it was to release her son from his cot. The secretary was supportive of parents as well as their children. This was an emergency for Jack and we needed to act very quickly. Everybody agreed that we had to support Jack's mother as well as her son.

In record time, the decision was made to give Jack a three day kindergarten program with a further two days in our training centre. Nothing else would work for Jack and his mother.

When I went to visit Jack's mother she was surprised by the news.

'I can't believe that you are going to help us so quickly. How wonderful. Now I can live like a normal mum.'

This incident convinced me that in the same way that children with a disability required access to education, so did their parents need access to a reasonably normal life. This was long before early intervention programs were made available to families in our national capital. As for Jack, well he was beginning a whole new life. His development at the centre surprised everyone.

When I walked into Mrs Viller's room one day a few months later, Jack was sitting at a table enthusiastically banging on some coloured pegs with a toy hammer. He could now use a spoon by himself when eating a meal sent to school by his mother. He had learned to stand in the first month and was walking between a chair and the nearest table within a year. It was remarkable progress for a six year old child whose mother had believed he would always be a baby. One day a few months later, as Jack ate the sandwich his mother had prepared before leaving for work that morning, Jack said his first word 'Mumma'.

Our work with parents of children attending the centre gave rise to many questions for me. In the beginning I really didn't under-stand why the diagnosis of disability was such a disaster for so many parents. Parents cope with babies and very demanding toddlers without much difficulty. So why was a child with a disability such a problem? I knew that many parents had been deeply disappointed by the diagnosis and felt that their expectations had been totally shattered. Do all parents want a child who will grow up to achieve whatever their hopes for that child are? And does any child with or without a disability actually live up to those expectations?

It was easy for me to ask the questions. Eventually families would show me how complex these issues are.

Visitors came to the centre every day. Some of the overseas visitors had been to other centres like ours and were instantly at ease with the children. I sometimes invited them to sit down next to a child and gave them a learning task to work on. Canberra had an abundance of visiting dignitaries, celebrities and diplomats. Wives with husbands in high office were particularly prominent on the schedule of visitors for the day.

One day the very observant wife of US Vice President Hubert Humphreys arrived with an entourage of extras. Later the American ambassador at the US embassy in Canberra organised a visit to the centre and afterwards his wife wrote a friendly, appreciative letter about her experience. She told us that sitting with a child at a table to develop his colour skills had been a very great pleasure for her.

Rolf Harris came to the centre twice and from the beginning had no difficulty treating our children like any others. He went through his repertoire of: *Tie me Kangaroo Down Sport* and the very popular *I'm Jake the peg ... With my extra leg ...* The children loved him and joined in the singing with gusto. He was totally at ease with the children and invited some of them to join him on the makeshift stage.

Celebrities were part of what was expected in a charitable organisation. And we were glad of the opportunity to meet them. But there was a down side to working in a facility supported by charity. The coupling of disability with charity was constantly around us. The organisation was in many ways a fine example of philanthropy, with members showing a commitment to fundraising and using the funds to extend and maintain the facilities. As a charity, donations came from residents as well as many of the diplomatic embassies and service organisations in Canberra. The building, our salaries and the equipment we used were all made possible through donations.

After the first year, when it took ages before the donated cupboards arrived, there was usually enough money for most of the equipment we needed. But the cupboards had been donated by a preschool centre upgrading its own to be more accessible to their children. When the secretary and I first saw the cupboards, we were both disappointed.

'I hadn't expected to see that ledge,' she said.

I stood staring at the cupboards and worrying about whether any child in our centre would be able to lift anything over the ledge on the shelf without help from a teacher. And independence was our aim!

Charity meant we had to be grateful for whatever people were willing to give. Sometimes people donated discarded toys in the hope that we would be able to use them. A neighbour brought a set of wooden animals that had lost their coloured paint. A volunteer carried a box of tattered books into the centre. One morning a lady, with a lovely smile, handed me a wooden jigsaw with two missing pieces.

'Perhaps your children wouldn't notice that,' she said.

The secretary knew that children with a disability needed the best equipment to assist them to learn. But charity often delivered the worst. And who was going to be ungrateful when people intended to be kind?

A further problem was that people are more inclined to give money when the handicap is emphasised and spun out by the media. So charitable publicity tended to focus on the way handicapped children differ from other children rather than ways in which they are the same. I was convinced that this distortion of reality affected attitudes to the children. Many parents talked about their child as being handicapped and abnormal. To receive charity was demeaning for many of these parents and added to their stress.

Working for a charitable organisation also disadvantaged teachers. Preschool teachers in Canberra were reasonably well paid and unlikely to apply for a position as a teacher at our centre. We worked because we loved the job, but the salary was barely enough to pay for my accommodation.

When I visited a preschool in an adjacent suburb, the differences stood out. We didn't have the range or the quality of equipment available to the children attending regular preschool centres. Working for a charity meant lower standing as a teacher, fewer resources and therefore educational limitations for the children we taught. Our dependence on charity devalued the education we were trying to provide. Education was still not the right of childhood that it had been for other children in Canberra for a very long time. Without charity there would have been nothing, but the time had come:

'We need to push for integration into the education system,' I declared.

My strong views about children having access to education had been kept in check for more than a year. Now they were unleashed by the injustice of unequal treatment. My own experience had shown that children with disability had the same basic needs as other children. These needs could be met by teachers who assessed what they had so far achieved and then did whatever was needed to move them on to the next step. In this respect, their educational needs were exactly the same as for any other child. Surely every child, whatever their ability, deserves the opportunity to learn whatever they can.

I needed to talk to a friend. It was a Sunday afternoon and we were hiking on the slopes of Black Mountain. I'd discovered the Botanical Gardens on the lower slopes of the mountain soon after arriving in Canberra. After walking through the grounds of the university and venturing over the road, I suddenly found myself in a truly enchanting garden. These were the years before Black Mountain was opened to cars, but there were many tracks formed by umpteen walkers enjoying the native shrubs and trees.

Now my friend and I walked easily along those tracks, chatting about this and that along the way. My thoughts returned to the children at the centre.

'It's normal in any country in the world for there to be children and adults with disability'.

'Yes, it would be a very odd country indeed if there were none,' my friend agreed.

My thoughts were firming up as we talked:

'Governments should provide education for children of all abilities.'

Then out came my most pressing hope:

'The kindergarten children at our centre should have a right to be educated in a preschool centre run by the Department of Education. Just like the other preschool children in this capital city.'

Nobody I knew had disagreed with this sentiment and certainly not my friend on this lovely sunny day on Black Mountain.

But what about the planning authority and possible opposition from the private association for which I worked?

I was surrounded by friends in the public service and my hiking friend in particular knew how things worked politically in the capital. I laughed with relief when he said:

'There is a way to get over the obstacles to your plan.'

His solution came in the form of Doug Anthony, a man with blond hair and a pleasant face who at that time was Minister for the Interior. He told me the Minister had the power to make anything happen in Canberra, and everywhere else in the capital territory. I trusted my friend's opinion because he worked in the public service and knew the system far better than me.

It was time to start testing the views of those in the association. I needed to know whether they were opposed to a move to the Department of Education or not. The secretary of the association understood this push for educational integration. I suspect that her major worry was what would happen to me. When I talked with another member of the association about the issue he was adamant:

'If the kindergarten is taken over by the department, the association will be delighted to have one less responsibility to manage.'

Then, he added:

'But your training was not in the early childhood area, have you thought that this might be a bad move for you?'

I knew that there was a chance that my job would not survive the move:

'But that should not be a barrier to this decision.'

'Well then I'll be supporting the move – that's if we have any say over what happens.'

That was good, but I knew that the development officer would be harder to convince. Then again, maybe his views didn't actually matter now.

As Minister for the Interior, and therefore responsible for Canberra, Doug Anthony had been invited to open the new wing at the centre. It looked like the stars were aligned and our chance was now. When the day arrived, the secretary and I escorted him around the kindergarten. The activity areas had been set up as usual like preschools throughout the ACT. He asked numerous questions and listened intently. I talked to him about our programs and what we hoped to achieve.

By 3pm our time was running out; it was now or never. So I

raised the issue of access for our children to the preschool service in the Department of Education. He gave me that wry half smile for which he was known. He said not a word. Would anything come of our conversation? Well, he hadn't argued against it, nor had he said 'yes'. But something in that smile gave me hope.

There were a few speedy outcomes of that visit. The first came in the form of government funding. The association received a grant to cover salaries and decided to double mine immediately to be the same as any other preschool teacher in Canberra. With that, I also became eligible for a government flat.

Was this a first step in the process, or was it all that could be achieved? My integration mantra was firm. I wondered whether anything was actually happening down the road in Parliament House.

That year I learned that the wheels of government turn ever so slowly. It was hard for me to be patient, but friends insisted that there was no alternative:

'Christine you just have to get on with your life.'

'What do you mean? This is my life!'

My new government flat was a small bedsitter for which I paid a pittance in rent and enjoyed the privacy of living alone and cooking my own meals. It was on the top floor of a three storey building and from the window there was a nice view of Black Mountain and the more distant Brindabella range.

The flat became a social hub at the weekend. My friend John was living at University House and through him I found out quite a lot about what the university offered students. My decision to go to university was being continually strengthened in Canberra. However I knew it would be impossible to attend lectures and at the same time manage the demands of my job.

My friend Maureen was working at the Barnardo's home in an adjacent suburb and I called round there one Saturday morning

to take two children from the home into Civic to shop and have
a cafe lunch. The Barnardo's home was a modern brick house a
little larger than others in the same street. Neither pedestrians
nor drivers would have noticed any difference from the road. The
kitchen was the central hub of the home and the children liked
to hang out there even when mealtimes were over.

A nice youngish couple were houseparents at the home and
Maureen helped with the seven children who lived there at the
time. I knew that some of the Barnardo's homes of earlier times
had been unpleasant institutions for children to be. Much had
since changed and this was a very good home for children. I
wished that the intellectually disabled children still living in
institutions could live in a place like this. However, even these
children needed to venture out. When two of them jumped up
and down in excitement in the hallway I knew that they thought
it was a treat to be going with me out of the door.

Later in the afternoon, after shopping and lunch with my two
charges, I returned to my flat. The *Canberra Times* lay on the
table and I picked it up. It was so good to sink into a chair and
just read. I turned a page and there was a heading featuring the
National Capital Development Commission. My attention was
immediately drawn as this planning authority was now of interest
to me. The column included information about a school building program and there, in clear black type, was news that the
authority had approved a special school and preschool service
in one of the new suburbs. Hope was immediately revived. But
what was meant by a preschool service? Once again I told myself
to be patient. Or perhaps, more accurately, a friend told me to:
'bide your time.'

Back at the centre, another issue came to the fore. And we
could do something about this immediately. When parents came
to the centre on their first visit, they often unburdened their

feelings. Many complained that they hadn't been given enough information about available services by the doctor who had first told them about the disability.

Jack's mother hadn't received any information from her doctor other than a diagnosis of Down syndrome. So she had no idea what to expect of her son. Little wonder she had continued to treat him as a baby throughout the six years of his life. Where do we get help and information? It had been a problem for all the parents I met. One day, when we were discussing this issue, the secretary revealed that the association might be able to help. In her typical problem solving style, she said: 'The association was set up to help parents as well as their children.'

We sat down then and there to make a plan. GPs, paediatricians and specialists at the Canberra Hospital and in private practice were probably surprised when the package of information about the centre arrived. An invitation to see the centre was included. This worked well and many doctors accepted the invitation.

Of all our medical visitors, it was the paediatricians in particular who were happy to sit down on a small chair and talk to the children. One took a sheet of paper from a pile near the easels and drew very realistic animal shapes and asked them to join in. It kept two of the children interested until Mrs Grant called them away for their morning fruit.

Parents and volunteers also came to the centre to talk with the doctors about their experiences and one of these mothers discovered that a good way to engage a doctor in conversation was with a slice of her famous chocolate cake. It led to a memorable sharing of views.

Many of the GPs expressed surprise about the skills our children displayed. A paediatrician said that he would now be able to present parents of newly diagnosed children with a more optimistic view about what these children could do. And the mothers were keen to let the doctors know how doctors might help parents. One mother, representing the views of many more, said that she would have liked more information about services from her doctor. A GP disclosed that there hadn't been any such information in his own training. Then he added: '... it has been very good to see happy and engaged children in this centre. I will certainly be sending the parents I meet in my practice to see what happens here.' Talking together had helped us all.

When a doctor who had only recently set up a surgery in Canberra phoned a few days later saying: 'I wasn't contacted about your open day and would like to visit. Is that possible?' I hoped it meant that word was getting around.

There was a sudden influx in the number of parents of very young children with a disability being sent to our centre. This meant that they could meet up with other parents as well as teachers and we could help them with information, and suggest activities that would challenge their child at home. They would also be able to see for themselves what our children could do.

The terrible circumstance in which Jack was discovered lying in his cot at the age of six would hopefully never happen again in Canberra.

Throughout this project I kept wondering how long it was going to take before our children would be integrated into education. My impatience had been kept in check for so long.

At last, news came from several quarters that moves were under way to integrate our preschool with all the others administered by the preschool office in the Department of Education. No official announcement had been made but one day, when driving with a friend through the new suburb of Garran, we stopped at a sign showing that a preschool was being built on the same site as the new special school.

'But can I be sure that it's intended for the children at our centre?'

My friend looked at me askance.

'Look at the bricks and mortar; that should give you hope.'

I stood looking at the layout of the foundations for a large centre.

'These could be two large rooms for the children and the plumbing may be for children's toilets, and those three smaller rooms could be anything at all.'

'But maybe that's the kitchen and this could be a staff room and an area for specialists.'

My friend laughed at this sudden display of optimism. Yes, there did seem to be a very good reason for hope. Something was happening in the Department of Education after all.

These were the years when good news often came by post. An official letter arrived with an invitation to apply for the position at the new Malkara preschool located in the suburb of Garran. Then there was a letter telling me that I'd been appointed as teacher-in-charge. Our children were to be integrated within the education department. It had happened at last.

It was an emotional moment for me when I joined the regular Canberra preschool service and the whole kindergarten moved with me. It felt like the government had finally accepted that that our children belonged to the diverse population of Canberra. The children had been included in the ongoing plan for this city. And their rights were now secure into the future.

It was exciting. Children with an intellectual disability and their families had a preschool run within the same Department of Education and under the same conditions as all the other preschools. Integration had arrived in the national capital. Nothing had mattered more to me than this and it seemed right to celebrate over dinner with a friend.

By the next day I was wondering what was left to do in Canberra.

'So what can I do now?' I asked my friend as we walked through the grounds of the university in the late afternoon.

'I'm sure you'll find something to stir your passions, but I think it's unlikely to be me,' he ruefully remarked.

It has so often been casually made decisions that produced turning points in my life and at the end of two terms at Malkara special preschool another such decision was about to be made.

Chapter 6

a chance meeting

O n the second last day of a holiday with the family in
Melbourne I travelled into the city to buy a coat ready for
another Canberra winter. The train was 'stopping all stations'
so there was plenty of time to think. Perhaps I could visit Keith
Cathcart, the training officer who had been a mentor during my
training. Of course, in the days before mobile phones, there was
no way of finding whether he would be there. The train finally
drew into Flinders Street station. By then, the idea of a coat had
been set aside and I headed straight for the headquarters of intellectual disability services.

The trams created a sense of vibrant activity in the city, with
people waiting on the pavement and taking precedence over car
drivers at tram stops. I tried to walk quickly down Swanston
Street, but the footpaths were crowded with people. Soon there
was the unmistakable burr of an oncoming tram and just inside
its entrance I could see a group of uni students who were laughing and joking with the conductor. The drama kept me amused
for more than a block. I reached Grattan Street about the same
time as the students heading for their first lecture of the day. Will
I ever get to go to university I wondered?

Soon the gate leading to intellectual disability services building came into view. There were no familiar faces among the
strangers who strode briskly across the courtyard from one door
to another. So much had changed. After a decade interstate I
should not have been surprised, but now I couldn't be sure that

Keith would be in his office. I should have phoned. Suddenly, there he was at the end of a corridor. His hair was now white; shining like moonshine in the dark corridor. Perhaps he wouldn't even recognise me. But soon his face broke into a familiar craggy smile and he pointed to a chair in his office.

We talked for a long time about what had been happening in Canberra, Adelaide and Melbourne and then Lorna joined us. She was the senior advisor responsible for educational programs in day training centres throughout Victoria. I'd met her briefly when she visited our centre years earlier.

'Do you have time for lunch? Keith asked.

As we all ate pasta marinara at a cafe in Lygon Street, he said: 'We are soon going to advertise for another training advisor.'

'What do you expect the position to involve? I asked.

Lorna laughed: 'Only half of the centres in the state of Victoria and umpteen lectures on the course.'

This was the training course I'd completed years earlier and my interest was sparked as we talked. By the time coffee arrived it was clear that Keith wanted me to apply for the job. Out of the corner of my eye I saw Lorna had offered a rather restrained nod of her head.

Coming back on the train everything began to fall into place. I very much liked the idea of working with students on programs for children. And the position of advisor would allow some part time study at university. I also expected that the range of disability services would be greater in the very big city of Melbourne. Long before we reached the Nunawading station the decision had been made. I would definitely apply for this job.

As it turned out, Keith and Lorna also wanted me in the job, so everything was set to go. Finding a place to live in Melbourne became an urgent problem. After being independent for years, nobody was keen for me to return to the family home.

'I think I will have to find a flat somewhere.'

My brother offered an overly eager 'Yes.'

He was happy that his big sister would not be disturbing his homely peace.

In earlier years my father had sometimes expressed worry about my failure to marry and settle down with a family of my own.

'When are you going to find a man to look after you?' appeared to be the main focus of his concern. Now he couldn't have been more supportive in my search for an independent home. Over dinner, he told me he had seen flats being built on Drummond Street in Carlton on a site previously occupied by a run-down hotel. We called at the building site the next day and picked up some leaflets for buyers. By then I had enough money for the deposit. And the deal was soon sealed.

It seemed like no time at all until I had set up a new home. The flat was a ten minute walk from the disability services office at St Nicholas Hospital and even closer to the university. It all seemed absolutely perfect, but a worry was on my mind. While jogging around Royal Park one evening I started to think about Lorna. Of course Keith and I would get on very well, but my work would be with Lorna and I hadn't had much contact with her.

A basic requirement for being appointed a training advisor was to have been a practising teacher. I took the position previously held by Stella who had left her advisory position in our department to be a lecturer in early childhood studies at the kindergarten training college in Kew. Lorna also came from the early childhood area of education in kindergartens. I guess that was why there had been such a big focus on play in the centres.

My worry about Lorna had to do with the programs I would run for the older children during my first years in Melbourne. I had been determined to show that when children moved out of the kindergarten section, they were capable of doing very much more than play. But there had been no word of support for these ideas from the department. Visitors from other centres had been surprised by what they believed to be my radical ideas about including such things as number concepts, sign recognition and community awareness in the program. Lorna had said nothing, even though the opportunity was there. Her warm smile on my first day as an advisor was reassuring, but the potential for conflict was always at the back of my mind.

On my first day in the new job I sat in my office thinking a few things out. By then I'd become a person more likely to confront problems rather than let them lie. Either way, in this situation, there were risks to relationships. First, was the contentious issue of programs for the older children in the day training centres. I decided to raise this with Lorna when an opportunity came. There were a few other niggling issues too.

We worked for the Mental Health Authority and the inappropriate name kept grating on my mind. The public service seemed to operate like a regulated machine. Our separation from the education department was particularly troubling. My hope was still strong that the children attending centres in Victoria, like those in Canberra, would eventually be going to education department schools. Government policy would have to change to include moderately intellectually disabled children in education, but surely this would happen before too long.

Lorna had warned me that public servants like me were expected to support government policy, but I believed that it would be possible to push for a transfer to education from inside the department. I was determined to raise the issue as soon as possible. In the meantime I could work on programs for children in the centres. As to the children in this hospital, well I hadn't even seen any of them yet.

Lorna and I had offices at opposite ends of the corridor. After a few days she appeared at the door waving a folder and suggested we move to the staff room where there would be more table space.

'We need to divide up our advisory responsibilities,' she explained

I took out another book from the cardboard box I'd brought from home and placed it on a built-in shelf next to the window.

'Yes OK I'll come with you now.'

We sat at the table looking at a six-page document titled *Day Training Centres in Victoria*, with pens ready to make two lists.

By the end of our meeting there were ten centres in the city and another nine in the country on my list for visiting. Our selection of centres in the country was based on me being a car driver and able to use a car from the department's garage. Lorna travelled by train and some centres were off the rail routes and therefore allocated to me. She travelled to more distant places by plane, so centres with regional airports went on her list.

Responsibility for lectures to students in the training school was the next issue to be resolved. Here was my opportunity.

'What subjects have you been responsible for Lorna? I asked.

She mentioned language, movement, early development and learning through play. Then she went on:

'So I thought you may want to develop some lectures on curriculum development and programs for older children.'

My anxiety dropped away.

'That would be great!'

We both laughed, and mine was with relief. Then she said something that surprised me:

'Of course, that's one of the reasons you were employed.'

The meeting had taken about fifteen minutes. Our work with students would reflect our major interests: hers would be on early childhood development and mine would be on curricula development for older children. There was no conflict, only recognition of each of our strengths. Our easy teamwork had begun.

Once again I found myself working with librarians to get all the relevant literature from around Australia and overseas.

Back home my flat was my haven. There were many days when, after arriving home, I locked the door and simply enjoyed being by myself in my wonderfully light and pleasant space. My already very private balcony was crying out for plants. It wasn't long before some particularly hardy ones had spread their foliage over the wall and provided further seclusion. Pelmets had been fixed to the windows and an Indian style brass lampshade sent interesting beams of light around the room at night.

Family members visited almost every weekend. My sister Pauline had married at nineteen and was now pregnant with her daughter. My sister Honor had married at 18 and soon she would have three young boys to care for. So I became the unmarried over thirty year old sister, and was enjoying my role as Auntie Chris.

Chapter 7

The St Nicholas Hospital
controversy begins

I hadn't seen it coming in the beginning, but an issue was brewing in St Nicholas Hospital where we had our offices. In the 1970s this was a hospital for severely intellectually disabled children. Like the subnormality hospitals in Britain and mental deficiency institutions in the USA it had been set up as a solution to the 'problems' caused by intellectual disability.

On my very first day, the superintendant had told me that the children in this hospital couldn't be cured and were the most severely intellectually disabled children in the state. During the 1970s there were more than 120 children in the wards, and the average age was twelve.

Lorna and I used one of the hospital buildings as a base for our work in the day training centres. My friend and mentor Keith also had an office in one of the hospital buildings, but he had announced that he was retiring.

We had a celebratory party.

'Goodbye for now old friend,' I said.

'So you remember our first meeting when you were nineteen?' And his craggy face broke into a smile.

Keith had been there from the beginning of my career when I'd made a naïve but determined decision to try to get a better life for children with intellectual disability and their parents. Keith was in charge of intellectual disability services and there was much to thank him for. In this sad and emotional moment, a very big hug was in order. Then out of the blue he said:

'It's good that you are still making things better for the children.'

Then he picked up his bag and left.

Keith had always caused me to assess what I was doing. Now, without knowing it, he had done so once more. I sat in my office thinking. Was I really still achieving things for children? Or was I simply supporting a system that was bad for them? The children in day centres were still excluded from education department schools. And how long would it be before the children in institutions, like this one, could live in houses like the new style Barnardo's homes I'd seen?

I was a very small fish in a very large organisation. And in the 1970s it seemed that only the psychiatrists employed by the Mental Health Authority had any power.

By then, Jean Vant had taken over Keith's job as training officer and we were set to become good friends.

I walked daily between my office and the training school where Jean had her office and it was then that I sometimes saw what was happening in the wards.

One day while waiting for the lift, I counted twenty large cots in one of the wards. Nobody I'd spoken to had expected these children to walk and that is why cots were used throughout the hospital. Memories of the year I spent in an isolation ward as a child often lurked in the background of what I saw here. My own release from hospital had been delayed when it was discovered that after lying in bed for so long, I could no longer walk. Would these children even have the opportunity to walk? My mind buzzed with questions: Why are these children lying in cots in a hospital ward if they can't be cured? Do any of them want to rattle the bars?

It was now more than a decade since I'd first seen institutions for children as a student. Not very much had changed. Later in the day I stepped into another ward on my way to the training school. It had white painted walls and about twenty cots. No colour anywhere to be seen. At first glance the children looked like large babies. But I knew most were well over the age of five, and many of those the staff called 'babies' were actually in their teens. The children had little stimulation except what the ward attendants were able to muster after the feeding, toileting and cleaning had been done.

It was an hour before lunch and one or two children were lying in their cots; three children lay on a mat on the floor, several were sitting on commodes or chairs they were unable to get out of. One child was being carried from bed to a chair. Another was being fed by spoon. Never did I see anybody helping a child to walk, or speak, or to eat with a spoon by themselves. Their parents had undoubtedly been advised to place their child here in this hospital. But what happened then?

To me, coming from a family where children had always been given lots of attention, the wards of the hospital seemed awfully quiet. Children had to be fed, and then movement around the ward seemed to cease. I was the eldest child in my family and fifteen years had separated me and my young brother. So, at the age of sixteen, I had enjoyed encouraging my brother to walk by standing him against the wall and holding out my arms from a few paces away. If he flopped to the floor before reaching me, he put out his arms showing that he wanted to do it all over again. On these wards, there were far too many children for any one of them to be given much attention at all. Visits from parents and siblings were not encouraged, and rarely happened.

Was there any opportunity for children to learn in this hospital? They certainly couldn't get out of their beds to explore what they saw through the rails. If children are not given encouragement to learn, what happens to them? And was it happening here in this hospital?

Some people I talked to in the hospital believed that children with a severe intellectual disability were incapable of developing any skills at all. My own experience as a teacher in the day centres had shown that there was plenty they would be able to learn. I was sure that if they had been in Mrs Byrnes' group for severely intellectually disabled children at the day centre at Oakleigh, many would have been using a walking frame, communicating and developing some skills by now. They would also be smiling.

One afternoon I paused at the door of one of the wards before walking out to the car park. It was about 5 o'clock and each of the 20 cots with rails had a child lying in it. The day staff had already gone home and I guessed that the night nurse was at her work station already. I could hear sounds coming from the cots, so I stood at the door listening for a while. I'd been told that none of these children in the hospital could talk. So I assumed that what I was hearing was similar to the babbling sounds of a very young infant.

Suddenly, standing there at the entrance to the ward, I could hear two quite distinct tones of sound and thought they must have been coming from two different children. I listened intently, but couldn't hear any recognisable words. I wanted to hear speech and there was none. Why did the second voice stop when the first voice started up again? First came one voice, then the other. I looked in the direction of the voices, trying to connect moving mouths with the sounds. Two children were engaged in this duet of sound. They were having a conversation, but not in a language that I understood, and they were not even in adjacent beds. But they did seem to be communicating with one another. Could that be right?

This was a disturbing moment that filled me with uncertainty about the children in this place. Suppose some of these children had the ability to communicate among themselves and nobody knew that they could. Suppose they had the ability to walk and no opportunity to do so. Suppose they had the capacity to learn and didn't have a school to go to.

I arrived at the hospital the next day in a questioning mood. Surely some of the children in this hospital had the potential to communicate, to walk and to learn. But would it ever happen?

A nurse was standing waiting for the lift when I joined her on my way to the training school. I asked whether she thought any of the children would eventually be able to leave the hospital. Her answer was a very blunt 'No' followed by a question that went right to the heart of the problem: 'Where would they go?'

A friend and colleague who knew me said: 'You shouldn't allow your own isolation as a child to influence your professionalism.' But how could I rid myself of those memories, how could I stop the tide?

A spark of optimism still glowed in me. Ever since talking to Keith after my first visits to institutions as a student, I had wanted them to be closed down. Perhaps naively I believed that this could be done by reducing demand for residential care. That's what had driven me to try to provide parents with a better alternative in the day centres. And to believe that parents who had been given little or no hope for their child would one day see their child going to school like other children. Now I wondered how the children in this hospital could ever get an education. The medical focus in the hospital was a big barrier.

It was all very frustrating. If only these children were living at home and attending a day training centre, Lorna and I could easily have organised an educational program. That would have been part of our job. But they were not living at home. Who was responsible? Who was the culprit and who could we blame? It wasn't the parents who, with no assistance whatsoever at home, had taken the advice of a doctor to place their child at the hospital. Nor was it the doctors who gave that advice believing that it was best for the family. Who was representing the children in this debate? Surely the needs of families and children both have to be addressed.

I knew that government policy would have to change, but who had the power to do that? Old and outdated policies tend to entrench what exists so only a major upheaval, coupled with action by government, could help. Or so I thought. But I was wrong. The first big nudge towards transformation came in a most unlikely form.

Dr Dennis Maginn was the superintendent in charge of St Nicholas Hospital. He very sincerely believed that he was helping parents by providing a place for their child at the hospital. But little in his training as a psychiatrist could have prepared him for this job. In the early 1970s he employed a young female graduate to assist with our course for teachers and later appointed her as a play leader to organise a program for some of the children on the wards. It was probably a decision he would later live to regret.

St Nicholas Hospital had always been intended as a hospital and was unsuitable for anything resembling programs for children. Severely intellectually disabled children with multiple disabilities were not expected to do anything much at all, let alone be educated. When Kenny started to walk by himself, this problem was exposed for all to see. Kenny had found that by a creative combination of physical manoeuvres he could get out of the ward to the foyer. And then, wonder of all wonders, he was able to explore the doors to the lift. When Kenny found this place to have fun, his bright eyes and determined movement conveyed a message loud and clear: 'Nobody can stop me now!'

Kenny sometimes hurt himself during his adventures outside the ward. This was of great concern for the nurses who were considering ways to protect Kenny by restraining him. It was not uncommon for children in institutions to be seated in chairs they were unable to get out of. Restraint through medication was also used in some places. Kenny's exploration was a big problem for the doctor attending to his cuts and bruises. Kenny, on the other hand, was excited by his new found skills and looked as though he was very much happier now. He certainly laughed a lot more; even when the doctors were carefully tending his wounds.

Some of us thought that if Kenny had been in an educational program each day he would have been using his new found skill on safe equipment. Where else but a hospital would a child's development produce such problems? Everybody agreed that the hospital was an unsuitable place for Kenny. But all the other facilities were full. The doctor said that Kenny would have to wait for a place where he could walk.

Rosemary (now a play leader) often called in at my office as she went past on her way from a meeting. We called her Rosie, a name that suited her bustling disposition and pleasantly flushed face. She was a talented, creative and caring young woman with a strong sense of justice for children. She too believed that all children could learn and, like many of us, was appalled by institutional care and the lack activities for children. We all knew that because the children in the wards had little to do, this would reduce their development. It was Rosie who worked overtime on a program to help them.

At the end of each day, when children had been fed and put to bed by 4.30 pm at the end of the day shift, I sometimes spotted Rosie going from one ward to another. She was hanging up paper mobiles over their cots and putting magazine pictures of interesting things on the walls. The children now had something colourful to look at instead of staring at the white painted walls. I sometimes heard discussions between Rosie and the people in charge, and it was clear that some of the doctors and nurses didn't appreciate this invasion of their clean and tidy wards.

Rosie started to question the lack of development in the children on the wards. Was it because of the severity of their intellectual disability? Or was it lack of stimulation in the hospital? With three years of university sociology behind me, I immodestly felt tuned in to this dilemma. We knew that these children had not only been handicapped by their disability, but also by the deprivations they experienced every day. There were no educational programs. And where were the places to walk, play, talk and eat at a table like everyone else?

Rosie and I were united in our belief that the hospital had a huge handicapping impact on the children. But I knew that the superintendent of the hospital was unlikely to agree. Nevertheless, he gave Rosie a room in the hospital to run her program. She had about ten children in the play group. The children had been classified as profoundly intellectually disabled and the superintendent said that many had additional physical disabilities, such as cerebral palsy. Most people in the hospital believed that they couldn't be expected to learn anything at all.

One day Rosie invited me to see a group of children she called the Beanbaggers. I think she probably used this name, based on the type of seating they used rather than medical terms, because she didn't trust the tests used to decide the level of their disability.

I went up to the top floor in the lift, past the depressing wards with rows of cots lining the walls. A door at the end was open and I walked into a pleasant room with large windows of light. Children were sitting in brightly coloured beanbag chairs that accommodated their unusual movements remarkably well. The room was the lightest and brightest I'd ever seen in the hospital. There were brightly coloured wall hangings, shapes and pictures, every way I turned.

Rosie was working at a table with Annie who had been in this hospital for eleven years. The records stated that she had brain damage which had caused cerebral palsy and had left her severely intellectually disabled. Rosie wanted me to see what she could do. My job didn't include any responsibility for children on the wards, but I sat at the table with them. Annie looked to me like a severely intellectually disabled five-year-old. Her arms moved awkwardly, as though out of her control. Her eyes moved around the room without focusing on anything in particular.

Rosie asked Annie to do a quite specific task. I watched her slowly put her hand out in the direction of the equipment and, with some helpful support for her arm supplied by Rosie, she eventually succeeded in the task she was asked to do.

Rosie told me that Annie needed support for her arm because of her physical disability. Quite frankly I didn't believe that Annie was doing by herself what she had been asked to do. So I made encouraging noises about progress, in the pleasant but dismissive way sceptical people tend to do, and prepared to leave.

Then came a noticeable change between the three of us, but most obviously between Annie and me. For the first time her eyes met my own directly and her face showed the most deeply-felt feelings of frustration that I had encountered in my life. Annie started to make sounds that indicated angry feelings. I found myself expressing apologetic words for not taking her seriously:

'I'm sorry Annie. You have done so well to show me what you can do.'

The outburst subsided and her face relaxed into a glum and frustrated stare. She hadn't said a word, but I was left in no doubt that my apology was inadequate. Non-verbal communication can sometimes reveal very much more than words.

It was this face-to-face encounter with Annie that propelled me into an informal support group with Rosie. We wanted to assess what these children, who were believed to be severely intellectually disabled, were actually able to do.

The first meeting was held in my flat in Carlton. Jean and Dr Meg, a social worker, arrived along with Rosie. Soon we heard the heavy steps of Dr Roger Wales, a psychologist from Melbourne University walking up the staircase to join us. This informal meeting would not have been approved by the department, but we all knew that a very important decision was about to be made. By the end of the meeting Dr Wales had taken on responsibility for assessing whether the beanbaggers were able to read. Approvals had to be obtained and he needed to be meticulous in his preparations. His report would not be available for several months. In the meantime the centres in regional Victoria required all of my time.

Chapter 8

Parents, magical cures, and the beanbaggers

We expected teachers in the centres to work with parents. I knew that if we were to avoid any more children going into institutions we must all support parents with a child living at home and not just the overly busy social worker. This was hard to do on my short visits to regional centres.

The parents I met often wanted more information, and in the beginning I struggled to answer their questions:

How can I find out more about my child's disability?

How can I get her to sit at the table for a meal?

Is there an operation available to reduce the size of his very thick tongue?

Where can I get special shoes to help him walk?

Where do I get information about how to explain his disability to other people?

How do I stop him from walking all over his brother's home-work?

Where can I find someone to help with his speech?

Do you know any babysitters who can deal with children who have autism?

Is there a pamphlet you can give me?

And so the stream of questions went on.

On a visit to one of the city centres I found Jimmie's mother waiting for me in the foyer. When we sat down in the office and everybody, including the pet dog, had something to drink, she asked:

'Is there anything that can be done for Jimmie?'

This was a good opportunity to talk about some very good programs at the centre and I spoke enthusiastically about what the teachers were trying to achieve.

But she soon burst out:

'No I mean anything that will cure his disability.'

Although we talked until lunch time I knew Jimmie's mother was dissatisfied with what I'd said and was still bent on finding a cure for his disability. My information hadn't helped her at all.

Many so-called cures for intellectual disability were being proposed by people around the world. Some came from unscrupulous operators trying to make money out of vulnerable parents. These parents would pay any price to have their child transformed into the child they might become. Medicinal remedies were often proposed, but there were also some quite bizarre and dangerous procedures. Submerging the child in a hole of a certain depth for a set amount of time was suggested by a community leader in Melbourne; another variation on shock treatment perhaps? I was deeply suspicious about all so called cures and tended to see them all as magical. Sometimes it was hard to distinguish fact from fiction and I didn't have enough knowledge to either accept or dismiss the claims.

A strong contender as a cure was the patterning program proposed by Doman and Delacato, who had their headquarters in the USA. They had come up with an intriguing idea based on the theory that children go through developmental stages in crawling and then walking. That sounded reasonable to me. For those children who didn't or couldn't do this by themselves Doman and Delacato proposed that they should be physically moved through these actions and stages. I saw one child lying on a table while volunteers moved his torso and limbs through the recommended exercises. The child looked perfectly happy about all the attention he was receiving and it obviously wasn't hurting him in any way at all. But was it helping him and his parents?

The volunteers were often relatives, neighbours or friends of the family and they joined parents in exercise sessions running up to six hours each day. Parents didn't have time to do very much more than organise people on a perpetual roster before joining the exercise team themselves. The amazing claim was that children could achieve greatly improved development using this method. Of course parents were excited and filled with hope. Some even took leave from work and gave up their usual activities to give their child a chance.

After following the program for a while some parents did see an improvement. Some spoke about their child being more alert and interested in what was going on around them. I wondered whether this was due to the stimulating contact with the people who came to help with the program, rather than any effect of the program itself. But parents were desperate and the program gave them hope.

I asked myself: 'Why can't our educational and physical movement programs give parents hope?'

The hope of a cure had energised parents and my cautious views on the patterning method didn't help them at all. Families often pushed themselves to the point of exhaustion. If there was little progress, they often blamed themselves for their lack of persistence. The patterning program itself was hardly ever seen to be at fault.

The distress of mothers and fathers was plain to see. But there were no respite services and none of us could offer an educational miracle. To make matters worse there was a financial crisis in residential services and expansion had been brought to a halt.

Parents were no longer being advised to place their child in an institution because there were no places left, and no money was available to extend the buildings.

Perhaps everybody is vulnerable to claims for a cure. Cures offer hope, certainty and a sense of control, and the slow pace of learning through education is hard pressed to come up with an appealing alternative. I suspected that the main reason parents were seeking a cure was because they were stressed and at the end of their tether. And there were almost no support services to help them. From their perspective, only a cure could achieve what they needed. From my perspective, the unfurling tragedy of parents searching for a way to change their child meant that we were failing to meet their needs. If only we could give parents hope of improvement in their child. If only there were services to help them. But with two advisors, two psychologists and four social workers for the whole state I couldn't be very optimistic about that.

In the meantime, the controversy at St Nicholas Hospital was developing. Rosie hadn't made claims of a miracle cure for the beanbaggers. But she was convinced that these children, previously believed to be severely intellectually and multiply disabled, were more intelligent than anybody else thought. How do you test such a claim?

Children attending school can be regularly tested by setting questions and marking whether their answers are right or wrong. Intelligence tests require spoken or written answers. These children were much too disabled to do either. I hadn't heard any of the beanbaggers speak and many of them had little control over their hands or arms, so they couldn't possibly write.

Despite the difficulties, it was very important to test Rosie's claim that these children were more intelligent than people believed. Jean and I were keen that the children should be tested and Dr Wales and his team from the university were coping with what we knew would be a very difficult task.

While these tests were going on, Rosie decided that the bean-baggers should have a picnic day with members of the support group. Almost everybody loves a picnic, but we needed a place suitable for eight children in pushers. My friend John had come to Melbourne around about the same time as me. When the idea of the picnic was raised I was looking after his house on the slopes of Mount Dandenong at Kalorama while he was on study leave in London. So I suggested 'How about having a picnic in the garden of my home in the bush?' Rosie accepted straight away and the plan for a picnic went ahead.

We met at the house in Scenic Crescent and sat in the garden for a while enjoying the trees and the spectacular view down Mount Dandenong towards the distant city. Each child sat in a folding pusher. After a while we wheeled the children down to a shop on the tourist road. Spoons were miraculously produced by the shopkeeper for their ice creams. Then we sat under the gum trees watching a game of cricket at the Kalorama Reserve.

On the way back to the house we had to push hard down the mountain lanes. The pushers continually got stuck in the sandy grooves and the children laughed every time they were jolted in their seat. These children had never been in such danger, and they loved it! There were squeals of delight and excited waving of arms.

As we walked, I noticed that two of the children were trying to stretch out their arms to each other between their pushers. Their friendship was plain to see. Best of all, the children were laughing. And some of us didn't even know they could. Every one of these children had been diagnosed as being severely intellectually disabled.

When we got back to the house, Dr Wales started to read a story to three of the children and they looked at the pictures in the book and listened intently to the story. Lenny and Willy laughed loudly when the doctor dropped the book and almost missed his seating on the garden wall. From where I was standing near the back door of the house, the children looked like any other small group of children enjoying a story.

Meantime Rosie left Annie, the child she had invited me to see earlier in the year, and went to attend to children some distance away. I could see Annie looking intently in Rosie's direction and her eyes steadily followed her wherever she went. Suddenly frustration swept over Annie's face. She uttered the loudest most emotional cry most of us had heard. We all turned in Annie's direction, having been stopped in our tracks by her cry. When Rosie started walking in her direction, we all returned to whatever we had been doing. We all knew Annie had achieved what she desired.

Nobody who witnessed that scene in the garden at Kalorama could have doubted that Annie wanted Rosie as her very own friend. Later Rosie simply explained Annie's extreme reaction as a bad case of sibling rivalry. She thought that even though none of the children were related, sharing a ward had produced feelings similar to those of siblings competing for attention.

At the end of the day I had some deep thinking to do. Annie was obviously very upset when Rosie left her to attend to other children and nobody had any doubt that this was because she wanted to be with Rosie. Were these children severely intellectually disabled? If they were, the events of the day had shown that they were just as emotionally sensitive as any other child. They had expressed excitement, humour, friendship and pure joy. Three of the children had enjoyed a story. And one child had shown a deeply felt sense of being abandoned by Rosie. But the jury was still out on their intelligence.

Chapter 9

Annie rattles the bars

When I next saw Rosie working with the beanbaggers, she was using an alphabet board. The board was a metallic base for brightly coloured magnetic letters. These children were unable to communicate through speech, so Rosie thought that the board would allow them to answer questions by spelling out their answers on the board. I could see that Rosie was supporting each child's arm as they touched the letters required to form words.

Rosie believed that supporting their arm allowed a child greater freedom to move it in the direction they wanted. I acknowledged that this was a way of helping these children to learn to read and communicate if they were able to do so. But I was worried because any physical contact between her and the child was bound to arouse suspicion. People said: 'Is she influencing the child's response?'

That is why the children had to be tested. All of them had some form of physical disability and all had been diagnosed as being severely intellectually disabled. The question was, were they?

Dr Wales and his team had come up with a testing procedure they believed would work. The method was quite advanced for the time. It required every child to turn their head in the direction of a card on which a word spoken by a research assistant was printed. A different word was printed on a card at the other side. So if a child turned their head in that direction it would be scored as a wrong answer.

A video camera was set up to record what each child did. If the assistant called 'boat' and the child being tested turned their head to the right where the word 'boat' was printed, this was recorded as a perfectly correct response. 'House,' said the research assistant and the word 'house' was on the left of the assistant so the child was required to turn their head in that direction.

Any testing was going to be difficult. There was at least one problem for every child being tested:

How much control over her head does Jan (a child with cerebral palsy) have?

Has Cecil's eyesight ever been properly tested?

I knew the answer was: 'almost certainly not'. And how could children, who had never seen a boat, or even a house, be expected to recognise the word by which it was known. A child who had never been taught to read would be unlikely to recognise these words anyhow. My belief was that the children needed to be educated as well as tested. But they were unlikely to get access to education, unless they could prove themselves to be educable. This was a disturbing vicious circle, and I could only hope that somehow there would be a way through.

Despite the difficulties, when the results of the testing came out they were very interesting. One child, later revealed to be Annie, got several answers right and then treated the session as a joke by giving incorrect answers on every word from then on.

'What is going on here?' we asked.

Her unusual response was interpreted by Dr Wales as being deliberately non-cooperative. That meant it was most unlikely to have happened by chance in a child who didn't know the answers. I'd experienced Annie's angry frustration and now some of us believed that she might turn out to be very smart indeed.

The results of the testing definitely showed that all the children were capable of learning. In the end Dr Wales reported that the children had given some indication of an ability to read and to respond to quite complex instructions. He suggested follow-up testing of their abilities and appropriate educational programs.

Nobody known to me was confident that this would happen. Dr Wales was shortly due to return to Britain. Rosie was left to get on with teaching the beanbaggers in the only program available to children in the hospital at the time.

Time went on and Rosie was frustrated that the superintendant of the hospital was not taking her claims seriously. There were signs of conflict between Rosie and him. People increasingly spoke in whispers and a few started to take sides.

In the middle of this dispute I received a phone call from a high ranking colleague who I had previously regarded as a friend:

'You shouldn't be involved … you'll find yourself in trouble,' was the message. It was clearly intended to end my support for Rosie and the beanbaggers.

The conflict was bound to come to a head, and it did so in a quite spectacular way.

Rosie and I were sitting together on a bench in the hospital courtyard when she dropped a bombshell that would rock the hospital for years:

'Annie used her alphabet board to say that she wanted to leave St Nicholas Hospital and live with me.'

I was not at all surprised by this revelation because ever since the picnic there was little doubt in my mind that Annie wanted to be with Rosie. But the issue could not be so easily resolved for a child living in a state institution. Rosie, however, thought that there may be a legal way to get Annie released.

'I think that a writ of habeas corpus is the way to go,' she said.

This writ is a legal action through which a person who is 'imprisoned' can be released from unlawful detention. Legal studies was my sub-major at university but its application to Annie's situation in the hospital seemed novel to say the least. The idea quite took my breath away. Then I started to think, why not?

If Annie was able to convince the court that she was being imprisoned without cause and against her will in an institution, she would have a good case.

Rosie went ahead and made her big announcement that Annie, who by then was eighteen, wanted to leave the hospital and should be allowed to do so. Not surprisingly, this request didn't go down well with those in high-ranking positions in the hospital.

A formal letter arrived for Rosie. The superintendent and the mental health commission had refused Annie's request to leave the hospital. They said that the method used to obtain her request had not been established. I suppose they meant that the method of spelling out her request on an alphabet board while her arm was being supported was unusual. And nobody could disagree with that. How else could Annie express her desire to leave?

The conflict was now out in the open. And the beanbaggers became the focus of government and public attention. We wondered what the department would do.

There were claims and counter-claims, and opinions were expressed every way we turned. A committee of inquiry was set up to investigate claims about the children at St Nicholas Hospital. Its formal report and conclusion was in general favourable to the institution rather than Rosie and her supporters. Then a supplementary report by two psychologist colleagues of mine challenged the departmental claims that correct procedures had been used in gathering information for this report. The fight went on.

In the end Annie's request went to the Supreme Court of Australia. The big question was: Is Annie being unlawfully detained in the hospital now that she has indicated that she wants to leave?

Annie, like other children, had been placed at the hospital by her mother on the advice of the diagnosing doctor. Now her application to leave was causing a stir.

Annie had been three years old when she entered the hospital with a diagnosis of severe mental retardation and cerebral palsy. The superintendant was adamant that this remained a correct diagnosis. I doubt that any follow-up testing had ever been done. I knew that once a child had been tested as being suitable for a placement, they usually stayed there for the rest of their life. Earlier that year, we had twice asked for re-tests to be done on a child in a centre I visited, but that request hadn't seen the light of day. We had all initially trusted Annie's medical diagnosis. But we knew that it was based on the opinion of the doctor who conducted the medical examination before her hospitalisation. And medical opinions do sometimes turn out to be wrong.

A major problem was that Annie had used an alphabet board to instruct her lawyers by showing whether she agreed with their statement or not. The question being asked by some people was: Are these instructions to her lawyers valid or not? Did Annie really want to leave the institution and live with Rosie, or was Rosie making that decision and then influencing her response?

Those who knew of Annie's life at the hospital were a little bemused by the idea that she may not want to leave. None of the people I knew who had witnessed her relationship with Rosie, and had seen her on brief visits away from the hospital, could entertain such a thought. Signs of her happy contentment with Rosie and her partner Chris had been sufficient evidence for me. Now it was a court of law that would decide.

The effort made by the Mental Health Authority to keep Annie in the institution was a surprise to many of us. The legal and medical debate was quite extraordinary.

Now things were set to become even more amazing.

Because Annie was so small, a major point of difference between the two medical experts was about her disability in relation to her size. Why does size matter? It turned out to be absolutely crucial in the dispute about whether she had an intellectual disability or not.

Annie was much the same height and weight as when I'd first seen her two years earlier. She was described during the legal proceedings as having a body similar in size to a five year old child. Her weight was recorded as 35 pounds and her height as 42 inches. Everyone agreed that she was very small for an 18 year old girl. The question was why?

Both medical experts agreed that her diagnosis of athetosis was correct. But the medical superintendant believed that Annie also had a condition in which a type of dwarfing of a child's limbs is always linked to an intellectual disability. If his claim was correct then it would be argued that Annie could not have come up with an intelligent request to leave the hospital, and her case would fail. The other medical expert, Dr Phil, came up with a different explanation. If he was right then Annie's case may succeed.

The crucial question was: did Annie have the type of dwarfing linked to an intellectual disability or not?

I was uncomfortably aware that Annie's future life depended on the answer to this question. Would she ever be given a chance to live outside the hospital?

Dr Phil agreed that Annie was very small for her age. But what everybody wanted to know from him was: 'Is there any evidence of dwarfing?'

And then the vital words came:

'Annie's trunk, legs and arms are all well-proportioned and there is no evidence of dwarfing.'

There was a collective sigh of relief from many people following the case. So what was his conclusion? Many people inside and outside the court were anxious to know. Then his considered response came:

'... It is unlikely that Annie has the condition linked to an intellectual impairment.'

How did Dr Phil account for Annie's small size? He explained this as being probably stemmed from feeding problems. What did that mean? No explanation was given. I thought of Jack in Canberra being fed baby food from a teaspoon at the age of six. He too had been very small for his age. And what about all the teenagers like Annie in this hospital, also being fed with a spoon? Were their feeding problems a result of their disability? In Jack's case, he grew very rapidly after he began to feed himself at our centre. So would Annie do the same if she ever got to leave?

The argument against Annie's departure from the hospital had been shown to be flawed. There was some further support for Anne's intelligence from Dr Phil. He told the court that he had found that Anne's 'yes' and 'no' answers, using her eyelids and tongue, had been deliberate and convincing. This was an important back-up finding for those questioning the method being used by Rosie to support Annie's arm.

Shock for some and jubilation for others. The court case had succeeded. There was found to be no just cause for keeping Annie in the hospital and the mental health commission and hospital superintendent were required not to hinder her departure.

The media had been following Annie's case and as we sat glued to our television screens that evening we thought of the joy Annie would feel now that she could go home with Rosie and Chris. Having seen Annie's reaction to being separated from her friend on the day of the picnic in Kalorama, I was thankful there would be no sibling rivalry in her new home.

But this was an ongoing controversy and it was not quite over yet.

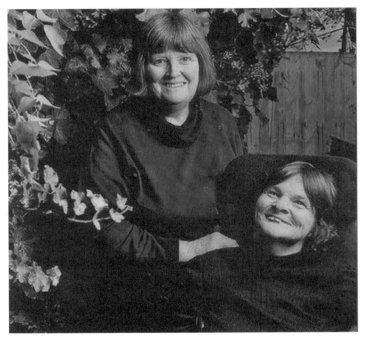

Rosemary Crossley and Anne McDonald.
Picture courtesy CP Blogs.

Chapter 10

A newsworthy crisis

Annie's intelligence had been questioned. But nobody was questioning the intelligence of the children in the day training centres. Once they were officially declared suitable for a centre, that's where they stayed. And the centres were already full. Newly diagnosed children had little hope of getting a place at their local centre and the waiting lists were long. Complaints about the shortage of places came into our offices daily.

'I wish we could just wave a wand and open up new places,' a colleague said.

It was a sentiment we all shared.

One day when I was at a centre in country Victoria, a mother arrived holding on to seven year Pete. She explained that he had been found to be suitable to attend the centre two years earlier. Pete eagerly looked around the room and then he called out 'hello' to the children working at the tables. He wanted to join them for sure.

The response from the supervisor was: 'Sorry, still no room.'

So Pete and his mother had to return home and continue their wait. Health regulations worked to reduce overcrowding in centres, but who was looking after the health and welfare of parents and children at home?

Exclusion of children with disability was a very common thing during the 1970s. It was happening all around Australia and also in Britain and USA. I knew that if Pete hadn't had a disability, the education department would be required to find a place in a school. There was no such requirement of the mental health authorities. The waiting lists at the centres were growing ever longer. Some children waited at home for years. This pressure on already struggling parents meant that the list of children waiting to get into the institutions grew ever longer.

A blanket of despondency was creeping over the offices of intellectual disability services. There were now about 45 centres in the state, with two more in process. Lorna and I couldn't cope with the centres in the city, let alone those in regional towns. But the most pressing problem was lack of support for families. On that matter, the social workers were barely controlling their anger and despair.

One day, as I walk along a corridor with a social worker, I found myself unburdening my frustrations about long waiting lists and too few advisors. In return, all I got was a litany of grief from her. The social workers were being pressured on two conflicting fronts. On the one hand, they knew that institutions were bad places for children; on the other, they knew that many parents couldn't cope and desperately needed help and support.

We all knew that when parents put their child's name on the waiting list for a place in an institution, it was often a sign that they had too little help at home. The consequences were all too predictable for children on the waiting list for residential care. It wasn't long before they moved into the most urgent category of need. To make matters worse, the people who knew best what was happening in services were restricted in what they were allowed to say. What could be done? Public servants don't criticise their employer, do they?

The social workers decided to write a critical report about the failing services. The report would focus on statistics gathered from all relevant branches of our department. I didn't know anybody who doubted that this was a crisis. We were excited that the social workers had decided to act. In the end it was the most comprehensive report I had seen.

When I went through the draft report with a colleague it was clear that every area of intellectual disability services was under enormous strain. I thought the report would be a political bomb-shell.

'They have to respond to this,' I told her.

Everything we had complained about was in that report. It described the poor support services to families as well as the impossibly large waiting lists. The inadequacy of our advisory service in having only two teacher advisors to cover more than forty day training centres was there in black print. There were statistics showing that the vast majority of children in the insti-tutions still had no access to educational programs at all. The chronic shortage of services was highlighted, and the statistical evidence of that was compelling.

The report was an accurate review of the problems, but would anything actually be done? We waited, but it seemed that a bunch of employees complaining about a crisis in services was not a sufficient reason to get anybody to respond. There were a few internal conversations. But absolutely nothing changed.

Momentum for action was also building outside our service, and Ethel Temby was at the centre of what was happening on that front. Ethel had worked hard in the development of the Kew Cottages Parent Association and later went on to found the Star Association on intellectual disability in Victoria. Our paths crossed many times over the years.

Ethel's baby Rowan was one of the babies I had seen in the nursery at Kew when visiting there as a student in 1958. Rowan was the name sister Eha called the baby who smiled at me when I leaned over his cot to talk to him. It wasn't until years later that Ethel told me why he was there in that institution.

Ethel's story was a sad and courageous tale of a parent who, in the beginning, and like many others, accepted the prevailing views about disability. During one of our conversations over the telephone Ethel told me her story:

'Soon after Rowan's birth I was told that there was a problem. A doctor said, "He's a mongol".'

She asked what that meant and was devastated when the explanation came:

'He'll be severely mentally retarded, capable of appreciating food and warmth but very little else – he'll be just a blob.'

Ethel asked, 'What can be done?'

'Sorry Mrs Temby, nothing can be done. In our view it would be best if you place the baby at Kew Cottages.'

They also told her to forget about him, but she never did. Against all advice, she and Rowan's siblings visited him frequently. Ethel was a founding member of the Kew Cottages Parent Association. She and others fought hard to achieve better conditions for all the children at Kew.

Time passed. When Ethel and the association found out that the child endowment money intended for the children at Kew wasn't being used to help them, they asked how that could happen. Every child in Australia and Britain was entitled to endowment. The children at Kew Cottages required much more than they had, so how could money intended for their welfare have gone astray instead of making their lives better?

Ethel and the parent association decided to raise the endowment issue at a public meeting.

The hall was gradually filling with people and some of those gathered knew about one of the issues to be raised. Some wondered why Ethel was sitting so far back in the hall instead of close to the speaker. They need not have worried. Ethel had learned that questions and answers were more likely to be heard from her position at the rear. She knew that it was an effective way to get the attention of Henry Bolte, the then Premier of Victoria, and for everybody to hear what she and he had to say. Her question was put ever so politely but it caused something of a stir.

She asked: 'Could the Premier please explain why endowment money intended for the children has not been spent on the children at Kew Cottages?'

The normally straight talking Premier Bolte didn't have an answer. But he did agree to speak with her after the meeting. When the meeting ended Ethel quickly made her way to where the Premier was standing. By then the meeting had dissolved into a social gathering and she wasn't confident that her message to him had been sufficiently clear.

The parents had been outraged when they found out that the endowment money intended for the children was going into government coffers for other purposes. The children didn't attend school and spent their days on the wards with very little to do. Did anybody care? Was it just another example of: 'being excluded – out of sight out of mind?'

Ethel feared that her meeting with the Premier might soon be forgotten. But, as always, she had a back-up plan: 'I'll write him a letter with the list of what the children need the money to be spent on,' she said.

She presented him with three pages of what should be done for the children with their endowment money.

Children needed:

Play leaders to run activities.

Everyone who had seen the children sitting around the wards, doing nothing at all, agreed with that. And Ethel's list went on:

Hairdresser, so that the children could have a haircut better suited to their individual features than the institutionalised basin cuts done by the staff on the wards.

The list ran into several pages of what the children at Kew needed.

Ethel's tenacity was strong and she was fast earning her reputation as a mover and shaker.

By now I knew that the government was more inclined to listen to parents than anybody else. I didn't yet know that Ethel was about to emerge as the number one advocate for intellectual disability in the state of Victoria.

Now, it was the lack of services and waiting lists that grabbed Ethel's attention. She knew first-hand about waiting lists. When she had wanted to bring Rowan out of Kew to live at home she had enquired about a place for him at a day training centre. The answer was: 'Sorry Mrs Temby, there are twenty-nine children on the waiting list for the centre in your zone.'

That meant that twenty-nine children would have to die, or move away, before a place could be found for Rowan. Would that happen this decade, next decade, or never?

Ethel did eventually find a place for her son. One of the centres I visited as an advisor was run by a Catholic order of brothers. One day I entered a classroom through glass doors. The teacher was organising children to take up positions around the room.

'Stand here, Rowan.'

Could this tall smiling boy be the teenage version of baby Rowan who was in the Kew nursery when I'd visited as a student? Yes, and Ethel was his mother. Rowan was now living at home and attending this centre daily. Our paths had crossed once more.

Ethel was now an advocate in the intellectual disability area and she was respected by us all. When the report written by the social workers came out, we had expected something to be done. But nothing had happened so far. It was frustrating for those of us who expected urgent action to be taken on this 'bombshell' of a report. We talked about how the shortage of services really needed media publicity. But there hadn't been nearly enough.

Fortunately, things were moving on another front. Ethel was working in her office at STAR, an organisation geared to advocating for children with intellectual disability and their parents, when the phone rang. Ben Hills and John Larkin were investigative journalists with the *Age* newspaper. Could it be that the much sought publicity was about to happen? The journalists told Ethel that they were doing research into facilities for the 'mentally retarded' and asked whether she was prepared to give them an hour of her time. Hills and Larkin drove to the STAR office to interview Ethel. Six hours later they were still there. Only a phone call at 6pm from the wife of one of the journalists brought this first episode of the interview to a close. This was going to be a big story.

There was a buzz of excitement in our offices. A few days later I picked up my copy of the *Age* in Lygon Street. The story we had been waiting for was there for all to see: the appalling overcrowding of facilities, the impossibly long waiting lists and the inadequacy of services. The issues had been graphically portrayed by the journalists.

During this publicity campaign the plight of children in the institution was canvassed by the *Age* under the banner of The Minus Children. It went on for many weeks. Some of us complained a bit about the wording of the title, but we knew that these journalists really cared. It was as though Hills and Larkin had opened the doors of the institutions to the public; for the first time *Age* readers caught a glimpse of the terrible conditions inside. As a result, the report written by the social workers in our department finally received the publicity it deserved. The information it contained, together, with information from Ethel and others, was out there in the newspaper for everybody to see.

I knew that publicity means very little unless readers are stirred to respond. Now I was about to discover that those seeking publicity have no control whatsoever over what happens next.

Mostly the reactions were good. Many readers were outraged by what they read in the articles and sent strongly worded letters to the editor. The series kept the issue in the minds of the people for months. We knew that there would have to be a satisfactory solution to this outpouring of public anger. There were plenty of ideas about better accommodation and facilities. But there was little agreement about what the solution to the awful conditions for residents in institutions should be.

One reader said: 'This is Australia, and the children in this country deserve a better life.'

But some of us wanted to know what was 'the better life' that these children deserved. Was it to stay in the institution, forever? A letter in the *Age* suggested that facilities at Kew should be improved and extended. Oh no! Other readers knew that the solution could not be to make the institutions bigger and better.

When I met a colleague in a corridor near the director's office, we could hardly contain our excitement about the success of the ongoing campaign. We chatted happily about the likely outcomes:

'Perhaps it will push the Premier to close down the institutions and build houses in the community.'

My social worker colleague saw the complexity better than me:

'We all want the institutions to be closed down, but what will parents do in the meantime?'

'Couldn't it be done gradually as the new houses are built and programs to families are established?'

In the end an activity centre was built with the proceeds of the Minus Children appeal. It meant that the children at Kew Cottages had space for activities that had not been possible on the wards.

When I read about the activity centre in the paper over break-fast one morning, my thoughts turned to Josh and Kip who had attended the day centre I'd taught at more than a decade earlier. They had tragically lost their mother, and then their friends, when they went to live at Kew. Were they enjoying their new facilities after spending fifteen years on the wards? We hoped so. And what about tiny Bennie, who had cried for his bottle on the day I saw him in the nursery? Now he would be in his late teens. So was he enjoying some relief from the monotony of his life in a ward? I convinced myself that a scheduled fortnightly visit to an activity centre would at least help.

In the mid-1970s many parents were angry about the shortage of residential places. I was constantly asking the question behind the long waiting lists: 'What can be done for parents who are unable to cope at home?'

If their needs could be met at home, then the waiting list would be greatly reduced.

Ethel had a meeting with the doctor heading our department about a letter she wanted to send to the parents of children on the waiting list. She explained:

'The letter will be about some options that parents of children on the waiting list might want to consider.'

Ethel left the office with permission to gain access to that long list of names and addresses. She was set to inform these parents about alternatives, such as day training centres. Our centres also had waiting lists, but we thought that perhaps this additional pressure and publicity would result in additional day centres being built. And maybe it would put pressure on the education department to accept these children into schools. Ethel's status as a good communicator and strong advocate worked again. A social work colleague posted the letters.

Things were happening unusually quickly. A meeting of

parents was called by STAR and of course Ethel was there. When somebody proposed that a rally should be held on the steps of Parliament House there was enthusiastic support for the idea. Around our offices we dared to hope that momentum was growing. Parents were angry and on the move. I knew many of the mothers with children on waiting lists and doubted that they would be able to attend. How could they possibly bring a child with difficult to manage behaviour into the city? And baby-sitters for such children were hard to find. But it was unwise to underestimate the determination of these parents. When I spoke to one of the mothers she said:

'Just wait! My mother has volunteered to help. This is a chance not to be missed.'

The day for the rally arrived. The parents mounted a protest like nothing seen before. Nobody could have anticipated that a crowd of 360 parents would turn up, along with representatives of all political parties. There were mothers and fathers with children in pushers and wheelchairs. Placards everywhere I looked, and everybody crowded together at the front of Parliament House. Anger and excitement swept through the crowd.

It was impossible for people to see everything that was happening. Fortunately the TV cameras were at work. On reaching home I turned on my TV for the evening news. The angry crowd outside Parliament House burst on to the screen. And 'yes!' the truly dramatic moment had been captured by the camera. A parent, desperately needing help, was presenting her severely disabled child to the Minister. The Minister was literally left holding the baby. The shocked look on his face on the television screen showed that he hadn't yet got the message which was strong and clear for many people in the crowd: 'Intellectual disability is an issue for the government and not just a family trying to cope.'

These were desperate parents and a response was required.

Under the scrutiny of the cameras the new Premier, Rupert Hamer, gave an undertaking to act on their issues. Parents had spoken out and the Premier had been given a strong message. The big test was: will anything be done?

Many frustrating experiences had dented my optimism. But when we discussed what was happening around the lunch table, most of my colleagues were hopeful: 'Parents may tread where public servants are ignored,' they said.

Months passed. Now journalists were asking questions. A journalist with an investigative intention rang Ethel to ask about progress. She told him: 'Nothing at all.' This incident had some of us believing that journalists were the most powerful people in the world next to parents.

The journalist had an important question for Ethel: 'What should happen now?'

Ethel had a pretty good idea about that. She had been reading documents sent to her by overseas organisations and was particularly tuned-in to developments in the USA. She was convinced that the issues facing us in Victoria were just as complex and broad ranging as those in America. Her answer was ready and clear:

'A committee like the one President Kennedy set up a few years ago in America.'

Yes, that's what needed to be done! Ethel believed such a committee would be most likely to sort out the complex pressures and come up with recommendations about the future organisation of services. This was the very best solution possible.

Things started to move very quickly. The journalist already had a draft of their story and a scheduled meeting with the Premier at 4 o'clock that same afternoon. The information from Ethel was the essential last step before that meeting. Everything was set to go.

When we picked up our newspapers next morning, the news we had been waiting for was there. The Premier had acted!

I sat with a friend reading the report and checking off the points one by one: A committee on mental retardation was to be set up to make recommendations to the Premier about what should be done. The committee would consider what to do about the institutions, the waiting list and the reorganisation of services. Relevant agencies, departments and groups would be represented on the committee.

When I later found out that Ethel would be representing parents on the committee, I laughed with relief. We could be optimistic that the recommendations to the Premier would be taken seriously, although we realised the report wouldn't be available for more than a year.

In the meantime things were happening on the educational front

Chapter 11

Schools open up

Although 'education for intellectually disabled children' had been my mantra since teaching in Adelaide I had achieved very little in the grand scheme of things. The children in Canberra had long since been integrated into education. But in Victoria, despite the efforts of many of us to push the issue along, nothing had happened for children attending the day centres run by our department throughout the state. Surely it was not too much to hope for? Why should a whole lot of children who were able to learn be barred from education department schools? And why should their teachers have to cope with inferior conditions for training?

The equipment we used in the training school was ancient. Lorna and I struggled to produce notes for students on an old fordigraph printer and we fell into despondency when our requests for new equipment were met with a cynical smile. There had been financial cut-backs for years and, just when we thought things couldn't get any worse, an announcement was made that the freeze on staff and equipment would continue indefinitely.

The inadequacy of what we were trying to do was there for all to see. One day, after venting her wrath on the printing machine for a while, Lorna mumbled:

'Let's hope that the courses of the future will be in teacher training colleges with proper funding.'

We all looked forward to that. We wanted our students to be trained in teacher training colleges. And we wanted the children in the day centres to have access to education department schools. At first I'd believed that it would happen.

Meetings about disability services were organised by various parent and professional associations during these years. Sometimes they were highly political in nature with the relevant minister in attendance. My questions at those meetings were often about our children being included in education department schools. It was a frustratingly slow process but we were determined to keep the issue alive.

Persistence did sometimes pay off. When the minister made an announcement about progress we interpreted his wry smile in our direction as recognition of the long drawn out process that had got us to this point.

Back in 1973, a law had been passed in Victoria giving the Minister of Education new powers to set up special education programs for children in institutions. And the minister was starting to use those additional powers. Education department teachers were being recruited to run classes for a few of the 'brighter' mildly intellectually disabled children in residential care. But most of the children in residential care were left in the wards without any educational program at all.

The day centres continued to be managed by private charitable organisations, with inadequate funding from the Department of Mental Health. The issue became a political football. The Federal Minister of Education described the administration of education for moderately intellectually disabled children as archaic. He wanted their education transferred from mental health to the education department. He suggested that the way to do this was to abolish clause 61 of the State Education Act which denied their access to free government education. He actually offered a $12 million grant for special education in Victoria if the state government (responsible for education) wanted it. It turned it down.

In 1975, there was a very hopeful sign from the USA. A law to open up education in schools to all children was passed by the US Congress. This had repercussions around the world. And we hoped that Victoria would not be too far behind.

A particular frustration in the push to give children in the day centres access to education department schools was that by the mid-1970s politicians usually agreed that it should happen. But it wasn't happening! Negotiations got stuck on details such as how and when? And there were legal issues as well.

When Lorna took twelve months' leave to upgrade her qualifications I became acting senior advisor. I was required to be 'at call' in my office for a good proportion of my time. Walking down the corridor one day I heard my phone ringing and rushed to the office to take the call. A voice said: 'You are being put through to the director'. I knew that meant an important announcement must have been made. I had been hoping for a message about the move to education. But it turned out to be a much bigger surprise:

'You will be pleased to know that funding has come through for four additional advisers and we can start recruitment straight away.'

We had been requesting more advisors for five years. So I assumed that the extra publicity we had been getting recently had produced this sudden decision to recruit some more. But when I put down the phone, pleasure about the new advisors turned into another fit of despair. My goodness! Did this mean our advisory service to teachers was going to be further entrenched under the Mental Health Authority? Surely not.

It was, however, great to have the additional help. That year I visited half the day centres in Victoria and at the same time passed the university examinations for my degree.

While Lorna was on leave, Jean and I continued to work with students training to teach in the day centres. Many of the students were from centres with poor programs for children. They were sometimes surprised to find that they were expected to take subjects such as child development, speech and language, psychology, services and family work as well as music, art and curriculum studies.

There were no suitable commercial aids available in the '70s, but students designed and made some very creative ones of their own. We sometimes had displays on long tables, stretching from one door to the next. Every year, there were some students who were eager to learn and others who were not. Some wouldn't have been able to get into regular teacher training, and others would have been outstanding in any course they chose.

The next morning I heard raised voices coming from the room where we poured our morning cup of tea. Rumours of change move ever so quickly and the day before we were all on alert. Something was about to happen, but nobody knew exactly what.

Through the open door I could see a newspaper spread over the table. I walked into the room and a colleague said:

'Have you seen the news Chris? The children in the centres will be moving to the education department'.

Once again we had been informed by a journalist. But at long last, the transfer to education was set to begin.

The children who had previously attended the forty-seven day training centres scattered around the state would now go to special developmental schools run by the education department. In some cases the building would be transferred. In some places a new building would be built on another site. The official notice informed us that 'everything will be negotiated'. Finally, in December 1976, the Education (Special Developmental Schools) Act was passed in Victoria. The children in the centres were at last going to an education department school.

Suddenly, it was all happening for us too. A new figure appeared out of nowhere in the corridors of the Mental Health Authority. Dr Lionel Murphy headed the teacher training program in deaf education. This course had been transferred to the teacher training college at Burwood and Dr Murphy was set to become the first dean of the Institute of Special Education within the college. His inquiry was about whether our certificate course for teachers could transfer to the same college.

Dr Murphy's plan sounded good. There would be a graduate diploma in special education geared to children with hearing and visual impairment and learning, physical and intellectual disability. Our two-year certificate course for teachers could be transferred to the college and retained as a course for as long as it was required. It was an ideal arrangement from my point of view.

I certainly wanted to continue to work in education. But I'd heard whispers that the committee advising the Premier would be pushing for a broad range of reforms in services. That meant people would have to be trained for those new services. I was caught up in the excitement of it all. Here we were on the cusp of a new era for services. The future looked good.

Dr Murphy had a strong connection with the committee advising the Premier and knew the situation well. When he asked whether we wanted to transfer or not, my own reaction was a very quick, 'Yes'.

I had always expected to transfer to education when the time came, and that time turned out to be now. Everything that I'd hoped for seemed likely to happen.

Chapter 12

In and out of the institute

On my first day in my new job I drove out to the college feeling excited about better facilities for the training of teachers. The first thing I saw on entering the building was a new photocopy machine. After struggling with an old fordigraph printer for years, this was an early sign of a better place to be. The institute was a basically functional double storey cement brick building. I saw a staircase at each end of the long corridor, with a staffroom and endless offices in between.

Dr Murphy came down the staircase with Ray, who was an expert in Auslan, the Australian sign language used in the deaf community. There were welcoming smiles and handshakes all around. It was Ray who showed me to my office upstairs. Through the window, I could see a pleasant strip of garden that stretched from one end of the building to the other.

'This is a good place to have lunch if you don't mind a dozen pairs of eyes on you while eating your sandwiches,' said Ray.

Never did I see anyone sitting in that garden, but looking through the window at shrubs and trees often inspired me with new ideas.

There were many changes in tertiary colleges throughout Victoria during the 1980s and we experienced every one of these. The teacher training college became a state college with a far greater range of courses. Later, following the Dawkins Report in 1988, the universities amalgamated with colleges, including ours.

But these were developments still to come and in the meantime I continued to work with students in special education.

An initial outcome of the advice to the Premier was the creation of a course in community welfare specialising in intellectual disability.

'That's great,' was my immediate reaction.

The course was intended to train people to support families in the community. I had always believed that social integration was all about meeting the needs of families, so this was an exciting development. I knew there was a big need for graduates from a course such as this so I was very glad to be made its coordinator. But, after the first year, government funding became an issue and the course was threatened with closure.

'We have to save this course,' I declared with conviction.

Students elected a delegation to go with me to Parliament House in Melbourne to argue our case with Premier Rupert Hamer. I hadn't been so politically motivated since arriving at the college two years earlier. We arrived as a group and climbed what felt like a hundred steps to get into the building.

'Nobody in a wheelchair would have access to this House of the People,' commented Gina.

The Premier, who was often described as approachable, greeted us very formally. We would have to present our case well.

The course was very definitely needed by families, but would the Premier understand? By then I'd learned a lot about the stress parents had to cope with. First I put the case that supporting families at home was not only needed but would reduce the need for residential care. Bev, a graduate of the course, helped to present our case. She was keen to give an example of what the course had trained her to do. The Premier leaned back in his high-backed chair.

Bev described how a mother she visited was trying to cope with Alan a hyperactive intellectually disabled child as well as his brother who had nowhere safe to do his homework. She went on: 'When I first met her, Mrs Jenson was stressed and didn't know what to do. It was bad enough that Alan was such a handful but, to make matters worse, her husband couldn't get home from work until the children were in bed.'

Bev described how she regularly worked with Alan until everybody in the family had learned some useful ways to manage his difficult behaviour.

The Premier's expression gave nothing away, and he asked her to describe Alan. Bev said he was seven years old, as active as a two year old, and tall enough to be destructive.

'On one of my visits I saw him empty a drawer full of cutlery and then pull down the cupboard on to the floor.'

Bev went on to describe what she did to help.

'I was able to enrol Alan in a special toy library. Then I showed family members ways to prevent him from becoming overly stimulated by introducing things one at a time. Mainly I listened to Alan's mother and we talked about what might help'

Bev told us that the hyperactivity settled down. The space within the home was reorganised and her husband fixed a latch device to a bedroom door for homework. She said that there was no simple solution to all the problems, but the family were now coping reasonably well.

It was a star performance.

The Premier stood up and walked several paces. We sat waiting expectantly for what he would say.

'I will organise funding to extend the course for another year. But the college will need to find its own funding after that,' he declared.

Fair enough.

We left Parliament House, excited and in a celebratory mood and went to have lunch in a nearby cafe on Bourke Street. Later, while paying for our sandwiches, I was horrified to find that the leather satchel in which my papers had been carried was missing and probably still in the Premier's office.

What followed seems very surprising in the contemporary context of top security in all public buildings; particularly Parliament House. I retraced my steps to collect my bag and was able to walk down umpteen corridors and get all the way to the Premier's office without anybody checking where I was going. A secretary was sitting at a desk outside the office and she laughed when I told her my problem.

'The Premier has gone to a meeting, but it is OK to go into his office and get it.'

From the door I could clearly see my bag by the side of a chair where I'd left it. The disturbing idea of bombs being left in black leather bags had not yet been created.

Getting funding for a course that should help to make life a little easier for families was good. But parents were also on my mind for other reasons. And one of these led to an important decision for me.

I had always believed that the best way to ensure that children were able to live at home and go to school was to ensure that families were able to live a reasonably normal life at home. That's why I wanted to find out how parents could best be helped. That meant enrolling at university for a part time PhD. Parents would be my teachers for the next few years.

Parents had always been a major force in achieving better services. And nobody had been able to achieve more than Ethel, mother of Rowan. She was representing parents on the Premier's committee. She had also won a Churchill Fellowship the previous year and sent back a stream of information about some services in Australia and what she'd seen in the USA and Britain. A great deal of that information ended up in the report of the advisory committee to the Premier.

When the report finally came out, it included 137 recommendations for the reorganisation of services in Victoria. It was a comprehensive guide to disability services. I sat at a table with a friend checking each of the recommendations. Eventually my eyes lighted on what I had been looking for.

'Here it is. They recommend that as soon as it is possible to do so, residents should move from the institutions into more normal housing.'

It felt like a huge transformation was just around the corner.

'I wonder what these alternatives to institutions will turn out to be?' my friend said.

'Hopefully, similar to the new style Barnardo's Homes I saw a decade ago in Canberra and Sydney ... and look, services from birth to old age are detailed.'

One recommendation was more important than any other. The Premier had been advised to establish an Office of Intellectual Disability. The implication was obvious to many of those I spoke with. If the Premier took that advice, the connection between the mental health services and intellectual disability would cease. These children would no longer be regarded as sick and in need of hospitalisation. The director of the proposed office would then have the power to make the changes necessary to support them in the community.

'That's exactly what is needed,' I said.

It was a huge relief.

The much anticipated report was sent to the Premier and the next stage in the revolution of disability services in Victoria was set to begin.

Chapter 13

Previously excluded children go to school

By 1986 most of the children from the day centres had been integrated into education department schools. So how was it all working?

On a cool day in autumn I drove to a special developmental school in Melbourne's eastern suburbs. I knew there would be many children who had previously attended a day centre, so this was an opportunity to see whether integration was working for them or not. The brick building resembled many regular primary schools, but the principal singled out one particular room:

'This gets a lot of use,' he said.

I put my head around the door and looked into a small room with a table and chairs of different sizes.

'We use it for individual work and speech development.'

'How are you finding the move to education?'

'It's great. The facilities are better, we have more teachers and the children are doing more advanced work.'

'Did all of the teachers move from the day centre?'

'No, two went to other schools and two stayed at the centre working with adults.'

'Are the teachers who moved to education department glad that they did?'

'Yes, I think so, although they sometimes baulk at the amount of paper work they have to do. It hasn't been very easy to cope with a new system, but it's getting better all the time.'

We talked until her next appointment. Then she said: 'The student is in the room at the end of the corridor. She's expecting you.'

I walked down the corridor looking through the classroom windows along the way. Activities were going on in each of the half dozen rooms. No surprises there. In the classroom where my student was working I saw about ten children sitting at tables, each working with a piece of equipment. The student was sitting at one of the tables with two children. They were assembling brightly coloured number rods in different ways.

'Hello Chris.'

She saw me looking intently at one of the children sitting at her table.

'Do you remember Pete?'

Pete was the child I'd met when he came to the centre with his mother to check the waiting list. He had been eager to join the other children at the centre but had to be sent home to wait. Now he was attending this school.

'Did you know that Pete's family moved to Melbourne just so that he would be able to go to school?'

I looked at Pete who was concentrating hard. His head was slightly bent at an angle that allowed him to more clearly see the rods in the pattern he was creating. His lips were pursed in a determined effort to arrange them according to the lengths and numbers he wanted.

'Pete was unable to go to school for such a long time …'

'… but now he is making up for it.'

It was easy to see that Pete loved school – but would he ever overcome the huge gap in his schooling?

The next week, I went to a regular primary school where a few children from one of the day centres were in classrooms learning alongside children who had no disability at all.

'Place your paper with the red line at the top.'

A teacher was addressing about twenty six year olds all sitting at tables around the room.

At one table a tall boy with Down syndrome was sitting next to an aide. He didn't have a paper with a red line and therefore had no reason to listen to the teacher's instructions. The aide was keeping him supplied with other things to do. When I asked about his program the teacher showed me a list of teaching objectives. The list didn't include anything remotely involving other children in the class.

There were so many challenging integration problems where children were being taught together exactly the same thing at the same time and only the child with a disability was left out. There was no contact at all between this boy and other children in the room. Were they avoiding him? Or were the aide and her charge avoiding them? Or was it just taken for granted that this boy would be isolated from what was going on in the room? It was hard to know.

These were still the early days of integration and perhaps it was inevitable that this separation of the child with a disability from other children would continue for a while. In the prep grade a boy with multiple disabilities was seated at a table with a teaching assistant who was showing him a picture book. The rest of the group sat on a rug for a story.

I went outside, thinking that integration still had a long way to go even for children in the same classroom.

Out in the playground a teacher was with a group of children, including one with a hearing problem. No integration problems here. They were taking turns with a hoop and enjoying the game. But on the other side of the playground an eight year old I'd known at a day centre was sitting alone on a bench.

It was a mixed picture of inclusion. Was I hoping for the

impossible to believe that children can learn to be inclusive of a child with disability? And that the child who needs a bit of help will want to join in. Perhaps some children with disability need to be taught how to join in, and for this to be a good experience when they do so. Other children need to learn that including them in their activities is cool. In Adelaide, the children had shown me that group work involving a wide range of skills allows everybody to join in and learn. So perhaps the method of teaching used determines whether integration works or not.

I walked over to another part of the playground just as a mother came through the gate. She recognised me from my time at the day centre. Her enthusiasm for the move to education was infectious. Since the beginning of the year her son, Bon, had walked to school with a young boy and his sister who lived further down the road. Their mother was a good friend of hers.

After a while it was easy to understand why she was so enthusiastic. And why the walk to school with other children had worked for Bon:

'The children know him really well now and they all play together, even at the weekend. Bon does what he can do and then just watches what the other kids do. They seem to understand his lapses and enjoy teaching him what to do.'

Integration was a big issue in the 1980s. A major obstacle was that children who had previously been isolated from other children hadn't developed the social skills needed to fit in. Learning those skills would take time. Education, at its core, is about gaining knowledge and skills about the community and broader world we live in. Learning what is culturally required in the community is at the heart of successful integration. And, as I was soon to find out, this is the case everywhere in the world.

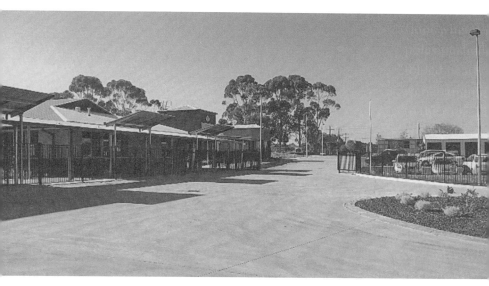

A special developmental school in Melbourne.

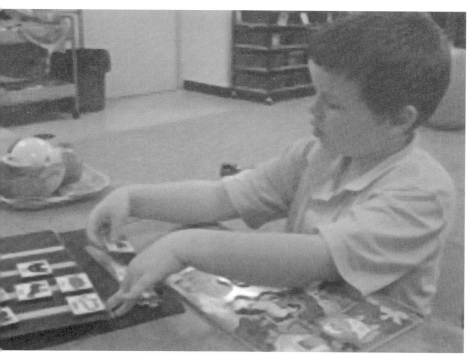

Concentration: a child in the classroom of a special developmental school.

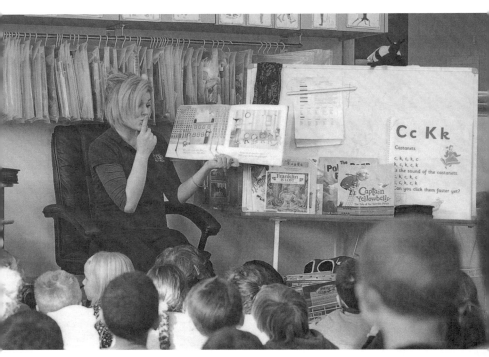

Inclusion support agency services ensure that all children can participate meaningfully and can be included, accepted and supported regardless of their ability and needs.

Photo courtesy of Noahs Ark.

Chapter 14

A normal life in Burma

A year or two after I moved to the Institute of Special Education, members of staff had been asked by the United Nations Educational Scientific and Cultural Organisation (UNESCO) to fill out a form with details of their qualifications and experience. A few years later I was very excited to be contacted by this organisation. My knowledge about what it means to be included were about to be challenged in a big way.

How do children become integrated in developing countries? By the time the letter from UNESCO arrived asking me to be a consultant in Burma, I had already been on a successful mission to Turkey. But Burma was a very different culture. I wondered how children with disability could become integrated into normal community life in a country run by a military junta. There was also the more basic question of what constitutes a normal life in a country with different cultural values and a different way of life.

My friend Bob promised to keep an eye on my house in Melbourne for the six weeks I would be away. Puddikins, my treasured long-haired tabby, would be fed and the bin would be brought in after the collection truck had been on Wednesday mornings. Soon I was on the plane to Rangoon.

Francis, the German UN officer in charge of the UN project in Burma was at Rangoon airport when I arrived. David, a consultant from Canada, was by his side. They stood at the far side of the Customs barrier waving and smiling as though they had known me for years. The photo in the UN folio had obviously worked.

After fifteen minutes of friendly conversation in the car, we had already begun working as a team.

Francis was definitely in charge. He was a tall man, clean shaven with a hair line receding ahead of its time. David looked like the university professor he was. His beard was tinged with grey below smiling and crinkly eyes.

Before going to my temporary home at the Inya Lake Hotel, the three of us walked through central Rangoon. There was an odd collection of red brick buildings from the British colonial period. The most compelling and amazing sight was the Shwedagong Pagoda with its one hundred metre high gilded stupa. Fifty tons of gold had gone into the building and, late in the day, when illuminated and with the setting sun on the stupa, the sight was breathtaking.

We walked towards what looked like a business district. A few cars were weaving between bicycles with carts attached and lots of people were walking. The women wore colourful sarongs and the men had sarong-like longyis tied around their waist. Everybody was busily going about their business, but I couldn't see anything resembling a shop. When I asked Francis where I could buy some teaching materials, he laughed and said: 'certainly not here.' His manner suggested that he didn't want to take the matter further right now. It seemed best not to say anything more on the subject. The question of where to buy things would remain a mystery for a while.

Francis dropped us off at the hotel. I was absolutely exhausted and slept for nine hours. My room overlooked the lake and the beautiful tropical gardens on its shore. From my window in the early light of morning the lake was a misty shade of pink. The palms stood like statues, not moving at all. In the distance I could see a Burmese man wearing a shirt with a longyi around his waist. He was looking out over the vast expanse of water. Francis told me that the Russians had built this hotel and there was nothing else like it in the whole of Rangoon. I took some folders from my suitcase and put them in the drawers of a large timber desk. It felt a little damp and the clothes I'd put in the wardrobe the previous evening were also damp. Despite the air-conditioning, humidity was getting into the room.

I sat on the only chair provided, gazing through the pink painted wall into outer space. So many new experiences. The previous day had been unsettling and I needed to think.

This was a country where democratic principles of government had been challenged and it was now ruled by a group of generals. This lack of democracy worried me. I knew that just like Australia, children with disability in Burma required educational programs. Because Australia had signed up to United Nations programs in developing countries, the Burmese Government had for some reason selected me from a list of UN consultants in special education. That was the job I was here to do. I calmed myself with the thought that the educational needs of Burmese children with disability were far more important than the politics of the country. I only hoped that politics wouldn't get in the way.

Walking out into the gardens for my usual early morning walk, I saw a few men dressed in longyis with shirts tucked in at the waist. They looked like gardeners and one stood next to a beautiful bed of flowers, looking out across the lake. I showed my pleasure, by waving my hands over the flowering shrubs and smiling. He nodded and smiled back.

My new colleague, David, was sitting at a table with two youngish men when I walked into the dining room for breakfast. They turned out to be working on an engineering project and had been in Burma for a month. I helped myself to fruit and toast.

The conversation turned to the Burmese military. Unlike in Turkey, I'd seen no men with guns on the streets of Rangoon.

So I assumed that the military junta was operating from government offices and the foot soldiers were busy elsewhere. The two engineers at the table put my impressions into a slightly different light. An army offensive was being conducted on the border with Thailand and refugees were beginning to cross the border. They believed that the lack of a visible military presence in Rangoon didn't mean anything at all.

'The military are everywhere you turn,' they assured me.

'Haven't you seen all the unidentified "spooks" hanging around Inya Lake?' added one of them.

Differences in culture and social freedom were challenging us all.

A driver dropped us off at the centre where I would be working for six weeks. I took a quick walk around the buildings. There was a workshop for adults with multiple disabilities and a schoolroom for children with an intellectual disability. The set-up was similar to the day centres I'd worked with in Melbourne, but the teachers had very few materials apart from a blackboard.

I saw a slender Burmese woman in a wonderfully colourful sarong, with a white blouse and black hair tied in a bun. She introduced herself in English as Lillian, the school principal, and talked in a friendly welcoming way about being glad to have me help her in the school. We went briefly into the schoolroom where a dozen children with intellectual disability were sitting in a semicircle around a teacher. Lillian said they were using an elementary school curriculum, but she thought it was unsuitable for most of the children in the school.

Frances was sitting in his office and I sat down with him and David to plan our work. We were soon sharing ideas about what it might be possible for us to do. Whatever we did needed to be culturally relevant. In my work as a teacher in Adelaide and Melbourne I'd consistently used curricula geared to life skills in programs for intellectually disabled children. So I was very keen to work with Lillian and her teachers using ecological inventories as a basis for this type of curricula development. The inventory is a listing of skills required in everyday life: those that every child with an intellectual disability needs to learn if they are going to be included in community life. It really didn't matter whether the setting was Australia or Burma; the technique used was exactly the same. Only the skills differed.

This sociological technique had been developed by Margaret Falvey in the USA and I knew that it was being used in schools and disability services in the USA, Canada and Australia. In Australia, I had taught students training for intellectual disability services how to use the technique. They had later used these inventories to teach people moving from an institution into experimental houses on the same site. The technique was found to be very effective in preparing residents for this new setting.

We believed that in Burma, as in Australia, if children could learn the skills required for life in the community, they had a better chance of being integrated within it. The skills would have to be those required in that culture. David was keen for me to work on this idea. Lillian agreed that learning the skills needed at home and in the community should be the base for what the children learned at school. So Frances made it a central part of our plan.

Lillian and I decided to set up a trial run for the technique by observing at a pagoda not far away from the school. That afternoon we walked through the gates of the pagoda and I stared at the amazing scene going on around us. There were several raised stone platforms with columns and ornate ceilings Steps led to each one. Inside, monks sat on the platform in red robes. A few children in trainee robes were sitting at their feet. Men women and children were all around. People left their shoes below the steps. Candles were being lit. Men sat in meditation. I needed Lillian to explain as we worked out the skills that children needed to learn.

In the end, the inventory of 'Pagoda behaviour' listed every step of the process, such as: Obeys rules regarding shoes; recognises planetary prayer post for meditation; knows how to approach Buddha image; knows how to offer flowers and candles; uses correct water pouring procedure; can recite common prayer.

For some children a much more detailed breakdown of each of those skills was required and Lillian and I worked on this together the following day.

'Why didn't I think of doing this?' Lillian said.

We laughed together like sisters who had just discovered something they both liked to do.

'Now,' said Lillian, 'every time a teacher or parent says that a child can't do something, I'll draw up an inventory of that skill so that we can all teach it step by step.'

What does a child with intellectual disability need to learn in Burma? What is most essential? Our plan had no hope of working unless the parents of the children attending the school helped and informed us. After David returned home to Canada, Lillian asked several families living in different neighbourhoods of Rangoon whether I could visit their child at home. I needed to find out what skills were needed for children to be more independent at home and in their community.

Soon I became accustomed to climbing the steps and ramps into houses built from bamboo and other natural materials. Lillian told me that most of these materials had been carried in from the surrounding area. The roofs offered good shelter but the front of the houses were often open to the elements. Privacy was not viewed as a problem.

In one home, family members were sitting on the bamboo

floor when I joined them. Clothing could be seen on bamboo poles pushed into the bamboo slats of the wall. Longyis were folded neatly on bamboo shelves. In another home, two shirts were hanging at the top of a bamboo pole that reached almost to the roof. This was a good way of getting clothing off the floor and out of the way. Ironing was done on the floor with an iron that was heated on the fire. Clay cooking pots and containers were standing in the middle of the floor. Cooking was done over a wood or charcoal fire. At night family members simply lay on a mat on the floor wrapped in a sarong. What a wonderfully simple life requiring so few possessions and no furniture at all. By contrast, how complicated life in many western countries has become.

Every home had extended family members. I learned that a daughter would usually continue to live in the home of her parents after marriage. Her husband simply moved in with his wife and the in-laws. Males were usually out in the fields every day or doing a job in town. So it was the women who worked around the home and spent most of their time there. Often an extended family of women were caring for children. And there were usually many children. Therefore the child with disability sometimes got lost in the rush. Some of the children tried to join in whatever other members of the family were doing. Others moved around on the fringe of whatever was happening. If food was being prepared, children in a family were expected to be involved in fetching and carrying as well as some of the food preparation tasks.

It occurred to me that Australian children, quite irrespective of whether they had a disability or not, would have great difficulty coping in this very different culture. And Burmese children would be similarly perplexed in Australia. Social values and ways of doing things are different in every culture around the world.

What is acceptable in one country may be considered totally inappropriate in another. Thus culture affects whether an individual is seen to fit in or not.

Parents wanted to explain and demonstrate the activities they wished their child to take part in. So I listed several skills required in Burmese cooking. One essential was how to prepare fish paste and cook curry using implements that were readily available. These would all be included in the life skills curricula. Self-care skills were important and I discovered that tying a longyi around the waist was one of the hardest things boys had to learn. Ordinary household domestic skills such as cleaning the floor by washing it had to be broken into very small steps. Children also needed to learn about health and safety and appropriate table behaviour. Elders had to be addressed appropriately and treated with great respect. It was considered most disrespectful to sit directly facing an older person. Language and communication with appropriate forms of address were also greatly valued.

The education program could easily be geared to skills needed in everyday life as long as parents, and possibly siblings, were involved. And Lillian, as principal, was keen to do that. First we needed to list the community skills and then draw these together with the numeracy and literacy skills the children learned at school.

But what about the skills required outside the home? Francis arranged for a UN driver called Wen to be my driver on the following Saturday. I spent the day going to villages and recording the life skills involved in whatever people were doing. It was the information I needed in order to work with Lillian on drawing up the inventories of skills. What other children learned easily, intellectually disabled children had to be taught. Breaking the skills down into small steps was the best way to do it.

Wen was a friendly Burmese man with a young family. I noticed that even though he had good skills in English he was very careful about what he said. One Saturday I asked him to drop me on the outskirts of a neighbourhood that was a half-hour drive out of central Rangoon and wait for me at the other end of the village.

Green palm trees were all around and bamboo houses on stilts stood tall against a bright blue sky. It was a pleasant scene. I wanted to see what children did at the weekend when they didn't go to school. I walked by myself along a road defined by a row of bamboo houses. A group of boys were playing with short sticks of bamboo in the sand. They laughed whenever the stick landed after they had flicked it into the air. I resisted the temptation to tell them about the risk of getting a stick in their eye and walked on. They were experts in stick-flicking and just playing and having weekend fun. An entry in my notebook reminded me that games and recreation were life skills that I should talk to Lillian about.

Through a gap between the houses I noticed a field of vegetables. Green vegetables were growing in rows. A young boy in a blue longyi was there with a man I assumed to be his father. The father was using a long blade to cut vegetables which the boy then placed in a basket on the ground. I wondered whether they were taking the vegetables home or to the market to sell. Seeing the young boy helping his father was a reminder. Gardening and field skills connected to the vegetable patch should also go into our inventory of life skills.

I turned back to the road, passing houses where men, women and children were sitting outside talking. In some homes people remained inside, sitting with arms hanging over gaps in the bamboo. The gap provided an open window to whatever was going on outside. Further down the road a group of women had gathered around a man who was bending over a large metallic container on what looked like a very large wheelbarrow.

Women and a few children were crowded around him holding clay, metallic or plastic pots. As I drew closer, all was revealed. The man was a water carrier selling his water to householders who needed to get it delivered to their homes. I stood watching this friendly social gathering. It was an opportunity for the women to talk to their neighbours and for children to play with their friends. When it came time for their mother to get their containers, the children were called upon to help. They were expected to place each container into position and help to carry them back home. They then poured the water from the container into the tank.

Here was another essential skill for the life skills inventory. So many elementary school skills were also involved. Money was used in the purchase of water. And number, measuring and communication skills were being used. I knew that many of the children at the centre would require each of these skills to be broken down into small steps; starting with one tiny step and then gradually building on this so that in the end a child would be able to do the whole task.

Wen was waiting in the car close by, so I asked him to try to find the village well. He knew exactly where to go. Much of life in Burma involved water so Wen had quite rightly got the idea that water was on my mind. On our way to the well he stopped the car.

'Do you want to see people using a water pipe?' he asked.

I looked in the direction he had pointed and saw a pipe coming out of a thick stone wall. Women and children walked past us carrying clay pots on their head and containers in their spare hand. I could see the water pipe had a very large tap. The skill was in turning the water on and off and then pouring the water from a larger container to the smaller ones. The children would soon be helping to carry them home.

We drove on into the heart of the village where Wen pulled up at the side of a narrow sandy lane near a large open area.

'The township well is down there.'

He sat by himself in the car. I walked down the lane, attracted to the vibrant scene ahead. People were moving around in rhythmic strenuous activity. Women in brightly coloured saris were everywhere. I walked over to a sandy mound and sat watching this colourful noisy scene. Mothers and their children used a timber pulley to draw the water. It took two people to manage the task. Then the water had to be poured into containers and carried all the way back to their homes.

Until then, my attention had been totally focussed on the well, but most of the activity was happening in a deep recess at the side. Here everybody was getting wet as clothing was pounded and plunged into the water. Every item was soaped into lather on a wash stone and plunged right back. A woman wearing a pink top above an ever dampening sari was washing her hair. Children played and washed themselves in the same recess. And some helped to spread out the longyis on the stone walls to dry. Children were laughing and enjoying the fun, but it was seriously strenuous work for their mothers and older siblings. And there wasn't much chatter between them until the washing was done.

Wen now had a clearer idea about what I wanted to see. On the way home he stopped close to a Burmese food store in one of the neighbourhoods.

'Look, there's a boy from the school.'

Kyi was standing at the door to the food store. I joined women and children crowding around containers of vegetables and a crate of fresh fish that had just been delivered in a cart. Money and goods were exchanged. Kyi was with a girl who was behaving like his older sister. He hadn't noticed me and was totally attentive to what his sister was doing. I'd been told that some of the children at the school were kept in their homes and out of sight of their neighbours, but Kyi was clearly quite comfortable in the shop. Even though he looked a bit different and his behaviour and speech also marked him as different, nobody seemed to be taking special notice of him. His sister showed the shopkeeper a note from their mother and soon their basket contained fish, vegetables and a couple of items from the shelf. Functional counting, money and measuring skills were being used everywhere I looked. A few signs were there needing to be read. Literacy skills were required. Kyi held on to the basket and his sister loaded it up.

I left the shop with a lengthening list for the inventory. What really pleased me most was that Kyi had been totally accepted at this neighbourhood store. He was truly participating in the everyday life of his village. I hoped that quite soon he would be able to go with a note to the shopkeeper from his mother. There were still many skills for him to learn. But maybe one day he would be able to go shopping without the help of his older sister. He would then be truly contributing to his family and doing what older children in his community did. It wasn't too much to expect.

I didn't see men with guns in Burma, but compliance with the rules set down by the junta appeared to be strong in the city. My time in Burma was before the 1988 political uprising which caused the military government to announce that a democratic election would be held. Therefore perhaps it wasn't so surprising that people appeared to be anxious about the political situation.

The mystery of where to get materials for the school still hadn't been solved. But after my second attempt to find out where I could shop for materials Frances said:

'Just wait a minute and I'll get Wen to take you now.'

'Can you take Chris to the market to get cardboard and a few other materials for the school?'

Wen seemed to be quite anxious as we drove away. After a while he drew into the side of a road.

'I'll park here,' he said.

'So where is the market?'

I couldn't see anything resembling a market.

'You walk down there. I'll stay in the car,' Wen said.

Sure enough, down a back laneway, there were items spread out on sheets. This was the black market. It was the only place in Rangoon where materials such as cardboard could be purchased. Apparently many materials were being brought over the Thai border illegally by carriers with large baskets who walked on tracks through remote areas to sell their goods in Rangoon. I think that the military must simply have turned a blind eye to what was going on. Wen wasn't taking any chances. He didn't want to be seen anywhere near the market that Francis had called 'black'.

Illegal carriers were taken for granted by the local population. One day at the school, a teacher asked me to write down the name of the skin cream she had seen me use so that she could ask a carrier to bring it from Thailand. Apparently there had been talk among the teachers about my skin being 'good for my age' and they put this down to the face cream I used. The thought of a barefoot carrier of a large basket containing, among other things, three jars of my own brand of skin cream illegally crossing the Thai/Burma border was quite amazing. But I later received a letter telling me that it had happened.

Wen's anxiety about being watched was displayed whenever I travelled with him. He was particularly agitated one day as we were driving past a beautiful part of the Inya Lake. I asked him to stop the car so that I could take a photo. He did stop, but insisted the photo be taken quickly so as not to arouse suspicion.

Aung San Suu Kyi, who would in 1990 win a democratically

conducted election in Burma, was unknown to me or my colleagues at that time. She had never been allowed by the junta to form government. More recently, when I saw on the news that an American had attempted to swim across the lake using home-made flippers and had reached her house, I understood why the lake had such great significance. I guess the lake has always made it harder for the junta to maintain control.

That evening we went to have dinner with two Burmese friends of Francis. They clearly made known their concerns about what they regarded as 'lack of freedom' in their country and their desire for democratic elections. We knew that UNESCO consultants should not engage in any form of political activity. But we listened carefully and did plenty of serious thinking.

By now there was an increasing urgency to complete my report. Lillian and I had already written up the ecological inventories as a basis for curriculum development. Now that my mind was focussed on recommendations, another major issue was starting to formulate in my mind. It concerned the isolation of children from services in Rangoon as well as other regions of Burma.

Many families had no means of getting their child to the school. This problem was troubling everybody. It meant that there was no means of addressing the stress experienced in isolated families and so many children were being deprived of any education at all. Lillian was also worried about how to get support to the teachers of children with disability in regular classrooms around Rangoon, as well as outlying areas of Burma. Transport to the school was simply not available.

The isolation of the school from the villages and regions where children with disability and their parents were living was a problem that somehow had to be overcome. But how? A possible solution sprang to mind one evening when I was sitting by myself in the hotel cafe.

While I was teaching in Canberra years earlier, a mobile unit had been set up by the preschool office to provide a service to families living in the newly developing areas of Canberra. On several occasions I'd worked with the teacher responsible for the mobile service when children with disability and their parents were involved. Since then many mobile services had been set up and were operating in states throughout Australia. First a mobile service was set up, then a regional service or school.

Could this be a solution to the problem we faced in Burma? Would a vehicle, or preferably a fleet of them, with appropriate materials and a visiting teacher, meet the needs of intellectually disabled children and their families? Would it resolve the problem of families being isolated in remote areas and children not being able to go to school? After mulling over the problem for a bit, it did seem to be a useful way of providing access to education and family support to people who had not previously had it.

Sitting there in the hotel cafe, positive thoughts turned into excitement. I asked a resident at the next table for a pen so that I could scribble some notes on a serviette. It took quite a bit of work to develop the design, but in the end my report listed twelve recommendations, including a mobile special education unit (a visiting teacher service)

The description showed how the mobile unit could provide services to disabled children and their families in townships where there was no special education facility and also serve as an advisory service to teachers in regular schools. The travelling teacher would be a link person to families and be responsible for checking their need for more permanent special education provision in outlying areas. Previously isolated children, families and teachers would then have access to specialised support.

Before leaving Burma, I had a meeting with people in the social welfare department about the visiting teacher service we had in

Australia. They were very interested. A key person in the department was particularly enthusiastic about the idea. Francis was coming to the end of his contract in Burma but he could see all the advantages of the project and he made a very determined effort to get everything moving before he had to leave.

A few weeks after I arrived back to Melbourne, a letter arrived with a Burmese stamp. I tore open the envelope straight away. The news was good. The Burmese were eager to get this project going. Two teaching fellowships and a UNESCO consultancy were being requested by the Burmese Department of Social Welfare. Already details of the type of vehicle and the spare parts required, maintenance, petrol and driver costs as well as the cost of the basic teaching materials required had been worked out.

Later I found that the mobile unit idea, based on the visiting teacher services in Australia, was being well used by children, their parents and teachers in Burma. The life skills curricula I had worked on with Lillian was incorporated into the education program in Rangoon and other areas of Burma. The techniques used in teaching for inclusion were surprisingly similar in both countries, and probably every country in the world.

In 2012 Aung San Suu Kyi, having been released from many years of detention and isolation in her own home, won a seat in what we all hope will become a more democratic government in Burma. She is now being included in political life in Burma after being kept out of government for so long. Life is looking better for the people of Burma.

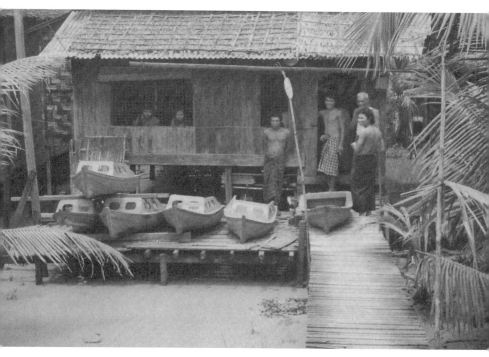

For this family their home was also their boat business.

Chapter 15

Getting over barriers

B ack at the institute, students gave me a look of disbelief when I said 'A child may be more handicapped by social deprivations than by their disability.' I had seen plenty of examples of this. I was thinking about Jack lying in a cot, with no stimulation, while his mother worked to support them both. She hadn't received any help with information about what her child with Down syndrome might be expected to do and was inclined to think that Jack wouldn't be able to do anything at all. When I first saw Jack he had been totally deprived of education and hadn't developed much over the six years of his life. And only a fraction of his slow development was due to his disability. Lack of services and support for this family was the biggest barrier to his development.

As for the children I'd taught in Adelaide, they had no interest in learning anything until given experiences outside the institution as an incentive to learn. And Annie, at St Nicholas Hospital, had experienced an extreme form of social deprivation until she was rescued by Rosie to become a celebrated co-author.

After a while students came up with some of the best examples of social deprivation. And they had good ideas about how it might be avoided. The story I liked best came from a student teacher. She described a youth leader's reaction when a father she knew called in at a club one day to enquire whether he could bring his son, Jamie.

'My son Jamie would like to come to your club,' he said.

'Oh, very good,' said the leader.

Then Jamie's dad, probably trying to protect his son, added: 'He has a learning disability, but that's unlikely to affect his activities at the club.'

The club leader baulked at the mention of Jamie's 'learning disability' and sadly shook his head.

'Sorry, we can't cope with a learning disabled child here,' he stated

That could have been the end of the matter. Jamie might have been sitting at home every Thursday evening and many Saturday afternoons while other children in the neighbourhood enjoyed activities at their club. Like many children with a disability all around the world, Jamie could have been excluded from an experience that would help him to learn. In his case the label was a potential barrier.

Thankfully a friend intervened by taking Jamie along to the club.

'I've brought a new recruit, his name is Jamie,' said the friend.

The club leader was quick to respond:

'Hello Jamie, welcome to the club.'

The youth leader didn't even know that his new recruit had a learning disability. So a very happy Jamie continued to attend the club regularly with his friend.

The students found many ways of dealing with secondary handicaps. But can people's attitudes to disability be so easily changed? Reactions to disability are in many ways similar to reactions to anybody else. Anybody that is, who looks or behaves differently. Or even people who simply don't have the same values as we hold dear. There are insiders and outsiders in every community and people find many ways to exclude those who don't seem to fit in. Laughter, taunts, ostracism, avoidance, ignoring and even an overly polite manner can indicate rejection.

The very worst type of rejection is when somebody who looks or behaves differently is then assumed to be a bad person. This sometimes happens in cases of disability. One such incident occurred when I was teaching in Adelaide. A young child had been sexually assaulted. The first person to have the finger pointed at him by accusing neighbours was a young man with the facial features of Down syndrome. I suppose he looked a little odd and had been seen looking through the railings at children in a local playground. What else did anybody need to know?

When neighbours accused this poor man of the crime being investigated, he was soon being treated as though he was guilty. Teenagers taunted him and one hit him with a stick, children called him names and some of their parents shouted their own abuse. Eventually, a perfectly ordinary looking man, who had never spent any time looking through the playground railings, was arrested and found guilty. Sadly, there was no report in the media about how the young man with Down syndrome had coped with the verbal and physical abuse.

The need to feel accepted is in us all. Rejection is an ever present threat. And sometimes it even happens in families.

For some children, having contact with people who challenge what has previously been taken for granted is a positive experience, and that was certainly true for me. My maternal grandfather was often rejected. People disapproved of his 'eccentricity'. He was shunned and avoided by family members and neighbours. Yet I looked forward to visits from grandfather. His appearance was unusual, and he was never very comfortable indoors. But my grandfather challenged my thinking about the world outside our front door.

'What have you got in your pocket grandpa?'

'Well, let me see.'

He plunged his hand into his pocket and rummaged around for

a while, prolonging my anticipation that something interesting was about to appear.

Sometimes he would take out a small clump of wild grasses, or a pebble picked up from the side of a lane. One day when I thought that the show and tell had ended, his hand went into his pocket once more. The fun was on again. This time a tiny twig from a tree was between his fingers.

'This probably comes from the cherry tree in the garden next door,' he said. See how the buds are ready to burst into blossom. I think that when you look at that tree tomorrow you'll see that the tree is covered in lovely flowers.'

One day he took out a small piece of broken glass and held it out in the palm of his hand.

'Look, maybe somebody broke a bottle of orange juice. But no, it's just the right size to be the thick bottom of a milk bottle.'

'Maybe the milkman dropped it,' I offered.

'Perhaps he had too many bottles to carry. Can you see any sign of old milk?'

'Yes, there it is …'

'Yes, now we know the glass is definitely from a milk bottle.'

At that point I saw my mother's smile change to a look of concern:

'Don't let her touch it,' she said. The next moment all the evidence of old milk had been washed away under the kitchen tap.

My grandfather was a great teacher. From him I learned that there were different ways of seeing everything, and that it is often a good idea to take a second look.

He once took me over to a climbing rose that I'd totally ignored many times that day.

He held a single rose above my head against an unusually bright blue sky and said:

'Look Christine, see how beautiful this rose is.'

I then saw for the first time what I'd failed to see before.

It was one of those significant experiences of childhood. Grandfather didn't fit in with the social demands of society. Neighbours were suspicious of his tendency to look overly closely at whatever he saw on the side of our lane. He wasn't accepted.

Eccentricity was one thing, but by the time I was ten I knew that being very tall or very short can definitely result in rejection. A favourite family walk during my childhood in Lancashire was to take the path through the cemetery past the grave of the tallest man in Britain. The grave was that of Frederick Kempster, who was eight feet four inches tall and had a career travelling around fairs throughout Britain. These fairs often had tents where people who were very tall or very short could be viewed by anyone prepared to pay money to the man at the gate. We are now totally sickened by such a practise. But at the Blackburn Fair I begged my father for three pennies to see The Shortest Lady in the World. She was described as being about thirty years old and less than three feet tall.

This woman had a home set up in the tent. I guess everybody in that long line of paying visitors wanted to see a person displaying her differentness. She was lifting a kettle off a miniature stove ready to make a cup of tea. Normal social etiquette was abandoned as people trooped around this miniature room staring, pointing, laughing and making loud comments: 'Look her arms are only as long as my daughter's doll.' A woman walking behind me said: 'I suppose she has to make a living somehow.'

Much later, my uncle told me that Frederick 'the giant' had also been forced to exhibit his differentness in order to work at all. Nobody had wanted to employ him.

Today the medical reasons for being very tall or very short are known. But, for my childhood friends and me, fanciful ideas overwhelmed rationality. As a very young child I ran past the grave of Frederick in fear of evil spirits lurking in the grave of the giant. And was always glad to reach the safety of my mother and father walking further down the hill.

Public exhibitions of human differences no longer exist. But have reactions to differences between people changed? Is everybody equally accepted? Or are some people still feared and rejected in our community?

I saw a documentary recently in which a psychologist claimed that the human reaction to somebody who looks different or behaves differently is a powerful force in us all. Even in very young children. These feelings are probably embedded within our genes. If that is true, then our initial reaction cannot be helped. It comes naturally. But after that initial natural reaction, what do we do next?

In recent years I've discovered that there is a big catch to achieving acceptance and a sense of belonging. It can never happen while people are isolated from the rest of the community. Mingling in common activities is what gives it a chance to work. This seems to be best achieved through a shared activity in which everybody has a role. People who work, play or study together usually get over their fear and reserve. That allows a sense of belonging to grow.

How will intellectually disabled people ever be accepted as members of our community if they are forever hidden away in institutions? That was one of the many questions we still had to deal with. We wanted to change a lot of things during the 1980s, and removing the barriers to community living was one of them. Belonging to the community was what it was all about.

The battle to achieve education for all children had been won. But progress towards abolishing institutions had stalled. Years earlier, the advisory committee had delivered recommendations about alternatives to the institutions. We knew that if the report was accepted, the residents would be coming out. But there was still no sign that it would happen.

I often thought about the children in Kew Cottages. Baby Benny with Down syndrome, who I'd seen in the nursery, would now be about twenty years old. Had he ever seen anything other than a series of wards in the institution? And the brothers Josh and Kip, who went into the institution when their mother died, would be more than 30 years old now. They would have missed out on anything resembling school after they were taken away from the day centre. Had they been upset about what happened to them? Like the two little girls who had clung on to me so tightly, they would have found it hard to tell anybody their feelings? They may have cried, they may have yelled and been destructive. But behaviour that stemmed from sadness or anger would probably have been ignored. It may even have been punished by the overworked attendants. Attention to the needs of individuals doesn't sit comfortably with congregate care. In a large facility with staff on shifts, who would have the time or inclination to deal with the problems of any particular child when so many others needed to be fed? Would anybody have even known or cared about the tragedy that had changed their lives?

As I sat thinking through the ongoing problems, my dark thoughts ran into a more positive frame of mind. Wouldn't it be good if residents such as Josh and Kip, now in their thirties, could move into an ordinary house. Perhaps they might enjoy gardening now they were older. A design for a vegetable patch, suitable for the house I hoped they would live in, sprang into my mind.

Was this more wishful thinking? Action on the report to the Premier was taking a very long time. And to complicate matters further, some people with power in the institutions definitely didn't want residents to move out.

Chapter 16

Carers fight on

It had been nearly two decades since I'd seen the new style Barnardo's homes. People with disability should be living in similar houses in the community by now.

A few years earlier, Ethel's son Rowan was the only child to be taken out of Kew Cottages and Annie had eventually been released from St Nicholas Hospital. A trickle has the potential to grow into a stream, and if it worked for individual children, we could hope for more. But was it working for Rowan and Annie?

I wanted to find out what had happened to Rowan after Ethel brought him out of the institution. Her story unfolded in her lectures to my students and then during our many conversations over the phone.

Rowan loved being at home with his family. He also enjoyed going to school. His trial leave flowed into permanent leave and Rowan didn't want to return to Kew. Ethel had been told by the doctor that Rowan would have a severe disability. But he did surprisingly well at the St John of God school. He hadn't previously had the opportunity to go to school, so he needed to catch up.

Ethel's story to students had us all enthralled. We sat in a circle around the room admiring her determination and appreciating the hope she inspired. Ethel told us that after a year or two in which Rowan made great progress, a party at the centre with children from an ordinary local primary school had got her thinking. As she sat in the sun watching the children, she noticed that

Rowan was playing with children from a regular local school, rather than his classmates from the centre.

'What is going on in his mind?' she wondered. 'Is he more capable than I was led to believe?'

Ethel was a trained teacher so she decided to set up a very practical test. That afternoon, on the way home in the car, she asked her son before each turning:

'Which way do I go?'

Rowan knew exactly which way through nearly a dozen turns. Ethel began to think that he should go to a special school for mildly intellectually disabled children run by the education department. Her views about her son's disability had soared through two official rankings of severity in three years. That night she wrote a letter to the education department asking whether Rowan could be transferred to an education department school. It took her a good deal of persistence but, eventually, Rowan did go to a special school.

Soon Rowan was walking a block from home to get the school bus without anybody escorting him to the stop. He was doing what thousands of children in Australia do every day. When I first saw Rowan as a baby at Kew Cottages, I would not have even dared to hope that he would later live at home and catch a bus to a special school. But he had, and he was loving school.

Ethel had to fight for everything her son gained and, because Rowan was already seventeen, the next struggle soon arrived. Ethel believed that children who learned slowly and had been deprived of early education needed to be at school longer. She pushed hard for a policy change that allowed these children to stay at school until they turned twenty-one. Again she was successful. Many teenagers, including Rowan, benefited from that change. They learned a lot during their later teen years and were then better able to cope with life as an adult.

Inevitably, Rowan and his friends soon turned twenty-one. Rowan had a party with his pals from school. Ethel decided to have a 'steam-boat dinner party' so that they could each choose the ingredients they wanted to cook. They chatted excitedly while watching prawns and other seafood being plunged into the bubbling broth. Yes, life was going well for Rowan. Nobody doubted he was having a normal life. But I wondered whether Rowan would ever live independently. What would happen when his mother grew too old to support him? As always, time would eventually tell that story.

Annie was the only other resident of an institution to leave for a better life at home. After she left St Nicholas Hospital she had greatly matured and made it known that she wanted to be called Anne. By then, Rosemary with her partner Chris and Anne had moved from a terrace house with umpteen steps, to a house that better suited their changed family needs.

Anne was now nineteen years old. Surprising changes were transforming her body and mind. She steadily grew in height and weight when she went to live with Rosie. We were all amazed by how tall she had grown – a gain of 45 centimetres. At one stage Anne held the world record for growth past 18 years. People were asking whether she had gained height and weight simply because she was more contented, or was it because of the availability of more food and the time needed with her friend and carer to consume it?

Did it help that she was now more active, was getting an education, and had a network of other young people around her?

Meetings about disability issues often provided an opportunity to meet up with friends. When I saw Anne and Rosie at one such meeting I was very surprised by the big change in Anne. She actually looked like a young woman in her early twenties. She sat with Rosie, displaying her agreement, frustration or boredom. Just like the rest of us.

But another battle was about to happen which would challenge Anne's desire to get on with her life. By now lots of people all around the world wanted to know what had happened to Annie. So in 1979, Rosemary and Anne were keen to jointly sign a contract for the publication of their story. Then a big problem arose.

Since going into St Nicholas Hospital at the age of three, and later while living with Rosemary, Anne's affairs had been in the control of the Public Trustee. She had been classified as an infirm person, which meant she couldn't enter into a legal contract. Once again, Anne had to run the gauntlet of the legal system.

I tried to imagine what it would be like to have to prove your intelligence in a court of law. How would I feel? How would my friends feel? How would Anne feel? But there seemed to be no alternative. Rosie had always claimed that this sort of testing infringed Anne's dignity, which was why Anne didn't like it. Everybody who had spent time with Anne knew that she had a will of her own and wasn't afraid to express it. But the courts require that people have a voice. Anne's friends knew that she had strong feelings about a lot of things. But she didn't have the voice to express it.

Any test that the court came up with had to show that Anne was capable of entering into a contract. This meant that Rosie's method of communication, using an alphabet board while supporting Anne's arm, would once again have to be put to a test.

At first, Anne was not inclined to cooperate with the testing at all. I imagined her sitting in the court with that look of frustration that I knew so well.

'Why are they putting me through all this again?' she would be wondering.

Many feared that she would respond against her own best interest as she still had plenty in her past life to be angry about. And, as I knew only too well, her frustrated outbursts couldn't be ignored.

The Senior Master of the court searched for a way of testing Anne's ability. Eventually he came up with what he believed to be a good solution. He gave Anne three words that he wanted her to spell using the alphabet board. This was done while Rosie was out of the room and had no means of knowing what the words were.

Anne was totally uncooperative in his first attempt. Frustration had set in deep.

'What if the case actually fails, what will happen to Anne then?' I wondered.

The master had to try to find a way to get Anne to cooperate. He took her aside and counselled her privately about the importance of the test for herself and Rosemary. Most importantly, he advised her to cooperate rather than dismiss the test as being beneath her dignity. That was the most persuasive thing he could have done.

When they returned, Anne spelt the word 'string' correctly and, instead of the second word 'quince', she spelt out 'quit' which the court took as a sign of her wit. I smiled, thinking this was undoubtedly what she had wanted to do from the beginning. When we heard the court decision, a friend said it for us all: 'Good on you Anne – you won your case and came out of that court room with your dignity intact.' Yes she had.

The Public Trustee was requested to sign and seal a certificate showing that Anne had ceased to be an infirm person and could take responsibility for her own affairs. At last, Anne could make decisions about what she wanted to do. And that included the contract with her publisher.

So, had Anne's release from the hospital worked for her? Well, she had used a legal system available to everybody outside institutions. And she now had a family life at home, an advanced education program, a part time job as a writer, and was set to receive an important award. Yes. Leaving the institution had worked beyond all of our expectations.

One thing I knew for sure: Opening up access and opportunities for children with a disability requires the efforts of a very determined advocate acting on their behalf. Ethel and Rosie are two such people. Rowan was very lucky to have his mother and Anne was lucky to have Rosie.

But should carers have to fight so hard? Should they have to strive at every turn to gain access to a better life for their son or daughter? Well, that story wasn't quite ready to unfold.

Chapter 17

One very big push

Tension was building in disability services. Despite my association with Rosie and Anne, I had always been a little uncomfortable with the St Nicholas Hospital saga. The focus on Anne's intelligence was a big worry for me. Rosie's argument (amended in the second edition of *Annie's Coming Out*) was that Anne's intelligence was the reason she shouldn't be in an institution. But many of us knew that institutions were bad places for anyone to live, and not only for those wrongly placed there because they were intelligent. Anne's release, therefore, as good as it was, hadn't helped the residents still there.

I often found myself in friendly but heated discussions with colleagues while we waited for meetings to begin. Some of us wished that a writ of habeas corpus could release all children into houses in the community. But now, we worried about whether it would happen at all. The authorities argued that all these children were intellectually disabled and therefore appropriately placed in an institution. To make matters worse, the government was proposing to build yet another one.

'Unbelievable,' was the only response to that.

Once again our frustrations merged into despair. It was taking such a long time for the policies on residential care to change.

In Australia, moves to get rid of the institutions had started more than a decade earlier. In the 1970s, Gunnar and Rosemary Dybwab, who were disability rights advocates from the USA, visited Australia. Several parents, including Ethel, along with a social worker and myself, met with them in the homes of advocates. A central topic in those meetings was the government's intention to build the new institution at Colac in rural Victoria. What we wanted were houses in the community.

I like to think that the project was delayed because of the opposition. But in the end, political priorities prevailed. The proponents of 'jobs for country folk' wanted an institution to provide employment in their country town. Thus we were faced with the reality of a new institution. When I met up with a friend from disability services we stood shaking our heads in disbelief:

'It's totally unbelievable that the government made that decision against the advice of so many people,' I said.

But on another front the situation was looking much more hopeful.

The committee advising the Premier had got a lot of people in the service thinking. The report had included Ethel's descriptions of some of the best agencies and services in the USA, Canada and Sweden and the Hester Adrian Centre in the UK. The report had been presented to the Premier way back in 1977. It carried a clear message that congregate care in institutions was bad for residents. By giving examples of places in the USA, it also showed that it was feasible to relocate residents into houses in the community. Some people had been asking how change could happen in large cities where so many institutions had been established and the medical system of care was so entrenched. Well, there was a surprisingly detailed response to that question.

The report recommended that an Office of Mental Retardation be established with the power to make these changes. Several recommendations contained instructions about precisely what the office should do. It showed why the institutions should be phased out, described better alternatives and outlined the way it could be done. All the pieces were in place for the changes to be made.

The report had bolstered our hopes. We had dared to believe that the transformation would happen soon. Why had there been no action on the report to the Premier? What was holding things up? More time passed, two premiers had come and gone and still very little had been done.

By the 1980s the mood for change was strengthening throughout disability services and students in our courses were excitedly involved in the new wave of popular thinking. Attention turned again to the overcrowded institutions. The calls for change were growing stronger and more strident every year. Many people around the world were writing about the need for change.

I was keen for the students to know about the work of Bengt Nirji, a Scandinavian who was the originator of the concept of normalisation. The essential idea was that services should closely resemble those available to non-disabled people in the community. But his writing was hard to read. Then a new writer on this subject appeared who became better known because he was so prolific, and who travelled around the world, even to Australia. His name was Wolf Wolfensberger and he was the person some of us hoped could push the international readiness for change into an unstoppable international movement.

Wolfensberger was working with the National Institute on Intellectual Disability in Canada. His philosophy of normalisation was about ensuring that people with disability had schools, homes and services equivalent to those used by other members of the community; along with social respect. In Australia, Wolfensberger's philosophy of normalisation had already been outlined years earlier in the report to the Premier. But Wolfensberger now had a presence that enabled him to bring to life what had been said in this and similar reports and articles around the world.

Wolf was a tall, thin man who many treated rather like a religious guru. By the time I met him, he had published several books and articles outlining his ideas. And this was an era when ideas had the power to move people to action.

The question being asked in disability services in Victoria was: 'Can this man achieve what the committee advising the Premier, and many others, has so far failed to do?'

We needed a charismatic leader who could get the government to act. We wanted the recommendations in the report to the Premier to be implemented rather than simply pondered upon, positively spoken about and then ignored.

On his first visit to Sydney, people from every state in Australia came to hear what Wolf had to say. My friend Tricia and I arrived in Sydney on an early flight. We shared a cab to the venue at Macquarie University and followed the paths across the campus. Judging from the number of people checking the signs to the theatre, it seemed certain there was going to be a big turn-out.

We joined a group of people going into the theatre to hear Wolf speak. There was tension in the room, but also rows of smiling faces and excited conversations. Some people simply waited expectantly. Many knew one another well. It was an audience of some who had a reason to hope and others who saw the speaker as a threat to existing services. As I sat waiting for Wolf to appear, I worried about whether this international guru would be able to deliver the changes so many of us wanted.

On stage Wolf displayed absolute conviction. His portrayal of disability services got everybody's attention. He was totally focused on his message and communicated it well. But was he the leader we all wanted him to be?

Some people found Wolf to be socially withdrawn and not at all keen to engage in ordinary conversation. When I joined a group of people drinking coffee after one of his lectures, I found they were anxiously wondering whether he would be able to do what was needed. They spoke about the quiet and unsociable side of his personality. Some of us thought he might simply have been exhausted by days of being on stage. We certainly didn't want this big chance to change services to stall. Nothing else had worked. Not pushing for change in meetings or in discussions with government ministers and their advisers, nor in talking to parents of children in the institutions or harnessing the enthusiasm of students training to work in services. In Victoria, the report to the Premier was sitting on a shelf somewhere with its most important recommendation apparently ignored. Everything seemed to depend on this man. He was needed to stir politicians into action.

We shouldn't have worried, but there was so much at stake. What most mattered to Wolf was his message. And that was really the only thing that mattered to those gathered to hear him speak. We all knew that disability services needed to be transformed. And here was the man who could push the cause over the line. Wolf was the essential link in the chain of action. And the time had to be right.

So, in its final phase in Australia, the reform movement was inspired by just one word; 'Normalisation' and one person, Wolf Wolfensberger.

There was a collective determination in many services to make the normalisation revolution happen. And government ministers were starting to take note.

Suddenly the word 'urgent' was being heard at meetings and in the media. Services in America, Britain, Canada and Scandinavia were also moving towards change. People everywhere were asking whether housing, schooling, employment and recreation for people with disability reflected the normal conditions of life in the community. The answer was clear: 'No not at all.'

In Victoria, the challenge was to disband five large institutions and give residents a more normal life. Policies had to be changed. But could it be made to happen?

Chapter 18

Transformation begins

At last it was actually happening! Disability services were changing everywhere in the western world. I saw this international transformation mainly through the lens of events in Australia, and more particularly in the state of Victoria. After years of being ignored by government, the pages of the report of the committee to advise the Premier had been turned by a new Premier, John Cain. The report became the blueprint that committee members, including Ethel, had always hoped it would be. However, not all the recommendations were accepted and many administrative and policy changes were required.

The first move was to set up an office on mental retardation. Hooray! That was the vital start to the process that would allow the changes to occur. In Victoria, Errol Cocks, a colleague of Guy Hamilton and a shining star of service provision in Western Australia, was employed as director. We were jubilant when we heard that he would have the essential powers to take services into the new era. It seemed that nothing could stop the transformation of residential services. And right now the state of Victoria seemed to be leading the way.

Nearly three decades had passed since I had unburdened my thoughts about institutions to Keith Cathcart. Now, while many people were opposed to their closure, all the excited chatter was about closing them down. It was a great moment in history for many people.

Ben Bodna, who was the first public advocate for Victoria,

swore to protect people with disability when they were being abused, assaulted, neglected or exploited. The idea of the 'least restrictive alternative' as a goal to be aimed for in services was part and parcel of what he wanted to do. We knew that institutions would fail that test. But everything depended on whether there was a better alternative.

Despite much opposition and concern from the parent association and the nursing union, the very first institution to close its doors before 1990 was St Nicholas Hospital. It was a bold move by new director Errol Cocks, and a strong statement. He believed that if residents who had been described as being the most severely disabled in the state could be relocated in the community, then so could the residents of all the other residential facilities.

Jan Harper, a fellow sociologist, had the difficult task of orchestrating the closure. She was project officer and manager of the St Nicholas Hospital project that had been set up to close this facility. One day, deep in thought, she found herself on the train travelling in the wrong direction, so challenging was the process of getting the children out. Later, Jan wrote a 200-page report about the closure of the hospital.

What follows is a summary of this report, sent to me by Jan. The full report has never been published.

The St Nicholas Project was the embodiment of the principle of normalisation. It aimed to provide an environment for residents more conducive to normal life routines, to facilitate more individualised and family-like care and integrate the intellectually disabled residents of the hospital into the community. As the first exercise of de-institutionalisation in Victoria it was inspired by the new director of the Mental Retardation Division, Errol Cocks, something of a guru among believers but a pariah for old school thinkers.

It was the first time in Australia, or elsewhere in the world, that the idea was put into practice to dispose of a whole existing facility and to provide the resources for re-housing residents in the community. Early on his watch, Errol Cocks proclaimed,

We must be prepared to re-allocate the resources that we are currently using in the area of retardation; that is, we must take the money that we are expending, the millions of dollars that we are expending; we must take the manpower, the thousands of people who are employed in this area; and we must take the physical environments in which handicapped people live; and we must be prepared to put them all together, to shake them so that they loosen, and then to use them more constructively and more efficiently (Patricia Lloyd Memorial Oration, 18 October, 1981).

In 1981, St Nicholas Hospital in Carlton housed 108 multiply handicapped residents in four wards. Although it had originally been for children, they had grown older and 25 of them were now over 16. There was a large component of non-contact staff, such as artisans, who did not work directly with the residents. The poor and outdated physical facilities and layout put great demands on nursing staff. One nurse described the morning routine:

"Come in at 7 am on the dot, strip 40 beds, put each resident in a wheelchair, make 40 beds in ten minutes, changing each whether wet or dry, bath as many as possibly by 7.30. You'd then line up all the residents in a semi-circle, one person would start shovelling in food at one end, another at the other end, and you'd meet in the middle. The other two staff would feed the more difficult eaters. After they had all finished you'd change them in the bathroom. Their basic needs were well cared for but there was no time for anything else."

Into this environment torpedoed the "Annie Macdonald Affair", in which Rosemary Crossley, made very public claims that resident Annie, as well as others in her communications group, had normal intelligence locked in a body that was unable to communicate. Uproar followed, the staff felt besieged and the claim led to an official enquiry. Into this maelstrom came the announcement of the St Nicholas Project.

The position of St Nicholas project officer was held for most of the project by me (Jan Harper). Several advisory committees were set up and met over the period of the project.

As in any exercise of dramatic change, the critics were loud. The most outspoken were the Kew Cottages and St Nicholas Parents Association. They said the project had 'left the vast majority of its direct-care staff grieving at the loss of their young charges that they had cared for, in some cases, for up to 20 years.' Some St Nicholas staff personnel were also very sceptical. They expressed concerns about whether the present standards of service in the hospital may not be maintained, and that promises made at the start of the project would not be kept. There was uncertainty, apprehension and mistrust.

The plan was, and remained, for 23 houses to be set up, each with no more than five residents, all of whom should have the opportunity to attend a suitable day service.

One of the factors ultimately contributing to the success of the project was that residents were assigned to houses in locations around Victoria as close as possible to their parents. If family members were not available they were placed according to friendships made at St Nicholas, their age group and whether a suitable day program was available to their needs. Naturally this required much consultation with nursing and therapy staff at St Nicholas, staff in the regions and parents.

There was initially considerable unease among parents. But

they were visited several times by social workers who helped to demystify the project for them. This relieved them of much of their apprehension. Changes were made to the intended placement of residents following these consultations. Deaths of residents and new admissions meant that changes had to be made right up until they had all finally moved out. Five residents from the 'communications group' of Rosemary Crossley were placed together in one house.

The uniqueness of the project meant its timetable could not be accurately predicted. We had to take into account new methods of housing multiply-handicapped residents, new local government approaches to permits and new methods of purchasing and instituting renovations. Further complications were created by newly emerging staffing models (including wages, conditions and training) new placements of nurses on regional teams and new methods of transportation and also financial arrangements. And then, of course, there had to be a re-orientation of thinking of day services to include this new and challenging group of clients.

All this meant that the starting dates had to be postponed a number of times. The move was initially proposed for July 1983 but was delayed until July 1984. After the final moves had been made there were 15 vacancies in the houses. These were filled by other intellectually disabled people in the regions.

All staff members at St Nicholas were given a commitment that they would be redeployed and were given the choice of being placed in another institution or, after training, being placed in one of the houses, provided they were thought suitable by regional staff. Staff training, for both nursing and unskilled staff, was seen as a vital part of the project.

The general consensus of the staff in the houses was that the new housing was successful. The day after the move brought this report from one of the houses:

The move proceeded smoothly. However, one resident has a seizure at 7.30 pm and was removed to hospital by ambulance. Staff handled the situation well and are keeping comprehensive records. The house is quite settled and staff are feeling good. Three parents have visited and been involved with residents. Some brought small furniture items and pictures. Morale is good.

Financial matters partly dictated the selection of St Nicholas as the first facility to be de-institutionalised. It was situated on a valuable site in Carlton and the sale of the site was considered crucial for the project. The sale had to cover costs of alternative accommodation. This created some hair raising moments for everybody concerned. The initial land valuation of $8m plummeted, there were zoning issues and some of the historic buildings had to be preserved. There were further complications with the many titles, so that the value decreased. The sale was finally completed in March 1985 for an amount of $4.7m, just covering the capital costs of the project of $4.2m.

So did the transfer of residents from a hospital into homes in the community work for residents and their family members? After the transfer a project evaluation took place, led by Dr David Dunt from the University of Melbourne. This focussed on measurement instruments such as the standards of housing, day placements, and residents' development, behaviour and health. In general, residents had gained weight, were more involved in activities of daily living, and were contented with their new lives in the community.

A resident whose disabilities meant lying prone on a trolley grew so much in the first few months that she needed a 30 cm extension to her trolley. A group who had their own swimming pool were revelling in the water and more than one had learnt to swim without assistance. A mother, whose daughter had never before made eye contact with her, now discovered that her daughter was able to track her movement around the room. Another female resident, who had always stayed in her own little world in the institution, began to walk up to, and hold hands with, the others in her house.

Parents were overwhelmingly positive. When asked how she felt about the move, one mother said:

'It's unbelievable. I cried and cried the day she moved. I'd repressed all the feelings I'd had when I put her in St Nicholas 10 years ago, and it all came back. I never dreamed she could live in such a beautiful place as this.'

Another mother said:

'I'm speaking out because I'm proud of where Aiden is. I can feel what other parents with children are going through now. I want to show them it is better. It's wonderful, so wonderful.'

In the beginning, the project was viewed with bemusement by many. But its completion showed, like a beacon, what could be achieved in the normalisation of life for intellectually disabled residents of institutions. Jason could have a bedroom to himself; Mary could show her family her new house; residents could enjoy music, put up their feet and relax at home. As one resident spelt out on her communication machine,

'I'm happy here. Thanks for everything.'

Change often carries painful consequences for those who have something to lose in the new arrangements. When Premier Cain announced that responsibility for intellectual disability services would be moved from the mental health area to be part of social welfare, the union representing the nurses in institutions went on strike. There were many issues to resolve. Nevertheless, the shift to community services happened. The most severely intellectually disabled children from St Nicholas Hospital were housed in the community and the dismantling of most of the other institutions began shortly after that. But it all took years to achieve.

Community organisations had always been the pioneering leaders in service provision and now new services were being set up, and already established ones were expanding. The Noahs Ark Toy Library in the southern suburbs had already been running for years. A service in the northern suburbs was beginning. And a few more disability services were springing up around the suburbs. The organisations previously responsible for the day training centres now focused on sheltered workshops and services to adults.

In Melbourne the advocacy movement continued to grow. Back in the early 1980s my friend Tricia had worked on a citizen advocacy program designed to support people with intellectual disability to live in the community. They needed a bit of help from a caring friend and Tricia's research, and her practical applications of it, showed how advocacy could work in supporting people in the community.

Self-advocacy programs were emerging. My friend Meg ran a centre in Middle Park, Melbourne, and from the beginning she and her staff were strongly committed to supporting people with intellectual disability to make their own decisions about their lives. This led to the setting up of a management committee involving clients and a change in the structure of the service. It was a significant milestone in the self-advocacy movement and the establishment of Reinforce; a self-advocacy group that achieved a great deal in Victoria. Subsequently, under AMIDA Accommodation Services, 50 per cent of the management committee were people with disability.

It looked like change was happening in stages, with one person's commitment to giving people with an intellectual disability the right to make their own decisions leading to a more formal arrangement where they had a strong collective voice. It meant that the people in these services gained some control over where they lived and under what conditions.

In Victoria during the 1980s intellectual disability moved from being seen and treated almost exclusively as a medical problem to being a social issue for community services.

Chapter 19

Coming out all over

Despite the jubilation, I was a little bit concerned about residents moving from the institutions into the new houses. Would they be able to adapt quickly to their new way of life? Most of the children I'd seen on the wards would be adults now, and many would never have attended school. Would they be able to cope in the big wide world outside? I knew many of them had been treated as though they were sick, incapable and totally dependent. So how would they cope in an ordinary house?

The children from St Nicholas Hospital would have the greatest challenge of all. When I last saw them most were unable to walk. They would have no idea how to use a kitchen, because they had probably never even seen one. Having a bedroom and a cupboard and wardrobe for their belongings would be a new thing for them to learn. In fact, the whole experience of having a house as their home would be new. It was all very well for us to think this was a huge improvement. But would they be able to cope quickly enough with the change?

The division of intellectual disability had established new services and wanted to find out whether the alternatives to the institutions were working. I was a founding member of the disability program evaluation unit at Deakin University in conjunction with RMIT, and glad to be selected to do some of the evaluations. If the houses for people in the community worked, almost everybody would be happy. Any problems would have to be identified and addressed.

Around the same time, I joined the community visitors (intellectual disability) program run by the newly formed Office of the Public Advocate in Melbourne. This meant that I could visit the community houses regularly and be an advocate for residents if they were not being treated well. We were glad that the community houses had been established, but some of us did worry about whether they would be the homely places we all wanted them to be.

I parked the car outside a house in an inner suburb of Melbourne. A voice on the phone had explained that two small single storey Victorian terrace houses had been opened up to make one. The facade of the houses hadn't changed at all, but I wanted to see what was happening inside.

The person in charge was a friendly youngish woman called Jane.

'I'll show you into one of the rooms, but you'll find most of the residents in the lounge,' she said.

As we walked around Jane described the layout of the home.

'There are six residents in this house and they all have their own bedroom.'

Jane opened the door of a room reserved for families needing respite care. It was a Saturday morning so most of the residents were at home. The respite room was empty and wouldn't be occupied until the following afternoon. Jane came to a halt outside a closed door and knocked.

'Are you there Bella?'

An indistinct voice said something about music, but we couldn't hear a sound. A young woman with shoulder length hair and dressed in a shortish dress opened the door.

'Hi we have a visitor and she would like to see your room,' Jane said.

'Come in,' said Bella.

She walked back into her room and started to talk quickly. I picked up about three words in every six. The tone of her voice was clearly showing pride in her belongings. She pointed to a picture of a horse on the wall and a poster of a place in the Grampians where she had recently been for a weekend. Then she sat on the side of her bed and chatted excitedly while patting her hand on the cover. Her prized possession was this brightly coloured bedspread with its prettily gathered edging.

Later, Jane explained that Bella and her stepmother had been to the market to get the material for the cover and had worked on the sewing machine over the same weekend. Bella's birth mother had died many years earlier, which was when she had to go into an institution for a few years before coming here. Her father had eventually married again and that had changed everything. Her step mother wasn't really required to spend much time with her stepdaughter, but it was what she wanted to do. Jenny told me that Bella's family enjoyed coming to her 'lovely new home' and quite often dropped by to say hello to their daughter. As we talked I learned the reason for Bella's earlier excitement about music. Her father had promised to bring her a new recording that very day.

We had always hoped that this sort of thing would happen. That's why residents had been located as close as possible to their family. This was definitely working well for Bella.

As I drove my car out of the driveway, a larger car with a pleasant looking man at the wheel drove in. His female passenger gave a friendly wave. I had no idea who they were, but hoped that it was Bella's dad arriving to give his daughter the music recording she was expecting.

The following weekend I went to another community house. It was early afternoon when the person in charge urged me to 'Come inside out of the rain.'

The door to the lounge was wide open and I could see a tall

young man dressed in jeans and a red and black cotton shirt sitting on a sofa with two others. They laughed together like any other group of friends. The person in charge told me that the tall young man had moved from an institution on the northern outskirts of Melbourne. Later, I went into the lounge room to find him.

'Hello, how are you all?'

'What's your name?'

'Chris,' I replied. 'And what's yours?'

The tall young man's answer was a short but clear 'Will.'

Will's new home could have been any house in Melbourne on a wet Saturday. He was wearing his favourite weekend shirt and preparing to watch the footie on TV. One of the young men sitting on the sofa had come from St Nicholas Hospital. His walking frame was at the side of the sofa. He didn't have much speech but he was obviously happy to be sitting next to his friends. When Will went out to the kitchen to get 'water, I'm thirsty', I followed to see what he would be able to do. He took a mug from the cupboard and easily managed to turn the tap and fill it almost to the brim.

'Do you like your new home?'

He nodded but looked surprised by the question.

'Would you like to go back to … [the other place]?'

'No.' He shook his head emphatically. 'I like my room.'

When he showed me his bedroom it was easy to see why he might be happy about having his own space. There were various items of football memorabilia from the Essendon Football Club on a shelf, and posters on the wall. A photograph of him and his friends working in the horticultural section of a sheltered workshop was on top of the shelf. The room was distinctively his.

Somehow it was his action in getting the water that showed how different Will's life had become. He had been thirsty. So what did he do? He knew where and how to get water, and he was able to get it for himself. Only those who had seen life in an institution would regard such an ordinary incident as wonderfully good.

In the kitchen, two other young men were clearing away some plates. A roster showed responsibilities for the day and a young man pointed to his name 'Bill.'

'That's me.'

'So that's why you are clearing away the dishes?'

'Yes that's me,' he repeated, pointing to his name. He gave me a huge smile. I took that smile as showing pride in his responsibility and a job he was doing well.

Each resident had their own bedroom with their own belongings in cupboards and their own clothes in their wardrobe. Some had photos of family members or friends. One had two birthday cards on a bench. Magazines and games were piled on a shelf. The music reflected the taste of those quite a bit younger than me. The house had access to an eight-seat bus which meant residents could be taken to the footie or other events at the weekend.

The transformation for Will and his friends was real.

Now, nearly a decade after intellectually disabled children were included in education department schools around Australia, the institutions were being closed down and residents were living like anybody else in the community. The only evidence required in our evaluation was what we could see with our own eyes.

When I asked the person in charge of one of the community houses what her secret was for such a happy household, she said:

'It's the individual attention we can give residents every day. They all have their likes and dislikes and, just like any household, everybody has to fit in. We try to make sure that everybody has what pleases them most'

'What sort of things do they show that they like?'

'Well, El likes to sit next to the window at breakfast so that she can see the sparrows picking up the bread crumbs she takes out there each morning. And Bev and Jay like to sit together at meal times. Everybody has what they need, and most of what they want.'

'I've noticed that the staff enjoy the residents and always address them by name.'

'We have a house rule that helps there. We try to ensure that residents get plenty of smiles of recognition from carers and always address each of them by their name.'

As we went through the door together she said:

'You know Chris, quite simple things like a smile and a hug can help to ensure that this place is not just a roof over their head, but their home.'

Exactly; my feelings entirely.

I had also noticed a few other positive things on my visits to this and other good community houses. Residents were being valued for what they each contributed to their home and they were being taught the skills they needed achieve this. They also had interesting group sharing and bonding things to do. Staff members respected and consulted with residents. They recognised individual differences, needs and preferences and used every available technology to find out what residents wanted and preferred. Equally as important, family members were made welcome and were encouraged to take residents out to family events and other activities in the community.

A memory kept flickering in the background of all of this good news. I had never forgotten the children I had taught at the school in Adelaide. How were they faring now that they were adults over 30 years old? Memories of children who had no reason to learn until they ventured out of the gate often crept back into my mind. Such sad and happy memories showed I had become overly emotionally attached to these children. Keith's advice had been that teachers should always take care to let go. Doing so had led to the crisis in my own life that had taken me to a new place, and a better educated me. But what had happened to these children? In Adelaide I had held on to an optimistic belief that they would have a good future. Now I wondered whether teaching about life in the community had all been in vain. Had these children been given the opportunity to move out?

The phone call from Pat in Adelaide was not unexpected. She said she had news about the children and would send details in a letter. I braced myself against the possibility that the news would be bad, and not what I wanted to hear.

'Do you remember Brian?' Pat asked.

I remembered him as the boy who seldom smiled and always wanted to be my helper in class.

'Some sad information I'm afraid.'

My body stiffened.

'I'm afraid he died from cancer at the age of twenty-six. But despite his earlier problems with depression, he had been living in the community for years.'

So Brian had gained a taste of freedom before he died. He would have had the opportunity to use the skills he had gained at school. He would have known what it was like to live a normal life. Sadness about his death was tinged with the pleasure of that news.

Pat also had some very good news.

'The two girls you asked about are living independently.'

I asked about Janet who had been a very pretty girl at school and had reduced class anxiety when she so easily befriended the inspector.

'Janet was able to get a job quite easily. She married and had children and I was told that she is a very proud mother.'

And what happened to Bobby, who had very few words, and Tommy?

'Bobby left the home after getting a job at a biscuit factory and Tommy was very successful. He also left the home and has never been out of work, even though his jobs have been many and varied.'

I asked about Michael who had Down syndrome and loved Pat's dog Pooch. The first words I heard Michael speak were 'Here Pooch.' In Melbourne I knew adults with Down syndrome who were living in houses. Two, with a bit of walk-in help, were sharing a flat together. But Michael was still there. Pooch the sausage dog had died at a ripe old age. I was glad to hear that there was now another dog for Michael to love.

The one other child that I very much wanted to hear news about was Billie. My throat tightened lest the news turned out to be bad. I talked on about this and that as a protection against what I didn't want to hear.

At the back of my mind as we talked I was thinking about Billie who, in my view, had shown no evidence of intellectual disabilty whatsoever. He had been such a talented painter. I remembered that he had been taunted with 'retard, retard' in his early school-ing before he became the star student in our class. Billie had been so very eager to learn about the world outside the gates. As I stood talking to Pat on the phone, I remembered how Billie had taken a map from our map reading class to try to get to Whyalla. On his return to school he had declared 'I'm going to be a police-man when I leave here … policemen know every road in South Australia.' What was the news about Billie? I had to ask.

'Tell me about Billie.'

It turned out that Billie hadn't achieved his ambition to

become a policeman. But he had found a job that used his map reading skills rather well.

'He became a truck driver with a company in South Australia,' said Pat.

'He would have done very well at that.'

'Yes, he must have been good because he has never been without a driving job. He married and had children and is living a normal family life.'

Now I could breathe easy.

'And does he have paintings in every room of their home?'

Pat didn't have that vital piece of information. But neither of us could think of a good reason why not.

'Thank you Pat – that's such good news.'

I was thrilled with the update on these children and even dared to hope that our life skills curriculum had helped along the way.

'We grew good people,' said Pat.

Despite the difficulties and deprivations of life in an institution, I was inclined to agree.

Although transformation was happening one further piece in the trail that produced these changes was still troubling me. And that had to do with parents and carers.

First, though, some issues were happening in my own life.

Chapter 20

A home in the bush, and a baby

T he decision to buy a country cottage happened quite spontaneously one Sunday afternoon while Bob and I were having
lunch.

I had first met Bob back in 1980 when he was recruited by
the new dean to lift the research profile of the institute. Bob's
arrival coincided with our planning for the International Year of
the Disabled Person in 1981. This was the year when Melbourne
disability rights advocate Rhonda Galbally convinced well-
known media identity Philip Adams, who had been officially
assigned the task of running the year's events in Australia, that
his plans could be improved if he let people with disability have
their say. The year will be remembered by many of us as the one
when disability access issues hit the front pages of newspapers
and television screens around the world.

In a dramatic event in Australia, a group of people who had
been diagnosed with an intellectual disability as children gained
unscheduled access to a professional conference. They presented
a charter of their right to decent treatment; including being
included in conferences such as this one. Suddenly, the audience
sat up and took notice of this amazing performance by people
who had previously been denied a voice.

That same year, Bob and I organised a weekend seminar at the
institute and co-edited a book on the conference proceedings:
Disability Human Rights and Law Reform. Bob was set to be my
very best friend.

And so the years passed.

I loved the location of my city house because it was amid a diverse and energising population of students and young professionals, immigrants and refugees. The mixture of rich and poor people was unusual for a Melbourne suburb and we enjoyed the vibrancy of the place. Bob had his own flat in the same inner-city suburb and we had both greatly enjoyed city life over many years. But the thought of escaping from the city for part of the week was attractive. I had always been happy and contented with my life and hadn't wanted to change much at all. Recently, however, the idea of a cottage in the country had been intruding into my usually contented mind.

On this winter afternoon in 1993 our conversation turned to my dream of a cottage surrounded by trees with a winding country road and 'definitely' there would have to be a fireplace suitable for burning the fallen wood for a fire. We had already shared some the delights of living in the country on holidays in various areas of Australia. As we talked, the idea of a country cottage emerged as something we wanted to do. That same afternoon we decided to find a cottage within easy driving distance of Melbourne. We were excited by the idea and within a couple of months had found the perfect place; Snook Cottage.

Among the Sunday visitors at a barbecue lunch were my sister Honor, her son and my nephew Tony, and his wife Lyn. The star was their baby daughter Maya. She was the first of a new generation in our family and was getting a lot of attention. My father was very proud of his great-granddaughter:

'Look, she has hair exactly the same colour as my aunt Edith,' he chortled.

He looked so happy to find that his genes had emerged in this wonderful new bundle of joy.

It was already past the usual time for lunch. People sat around the table waiting while bowls of salad were carried out on to the shady deck.

Honor could hardly wait to tell us her first proud grandmother story:

'Maya is such a wonderfully contented baby. When I went into the bedroom and looked into her crib this morning she was babbling away by herself without any sign of a cry.'

We all agreed that she was a very good baby, and Lyn and Tony were extremely lucky parents. They stood smiling at their beautiful baby daughter, their arms entwined.

Lyn said: 'She is such a happy, healthy baby and brings us such joy.'

Over the next two years, Bob and I renovated Snook Cottage to make it comfortable. It became a popular place for family gatherings and, if walls could speak, the joys and sorrows of our meandering extended family would be revealed. One such story carried particular poignancy for me.

In the meantime a whole lot of other families had their own stories to tell.

Chapter 21

Parents seeking a normal life

Way back in my very first teaching job at the day training centre, some of us had wondered how we would feel if told that our own child had a disability. We were rather biased on this subject. As we chatted in the staff room about the delightful children in our groups, some of us thought such a diagnosis might be accepted with appreciation rather than sadness. We enjoyed all our charges and were grateful for the warmth and joy they contributed to our own daily lives. But we never had to adjust to the impact of the diagnosis. Every afternoon we happily waved the children goodbye and went to our homes in the suburbs. We had made a deliberate decision to do this job. And we loved it. But parents had their own stories to tell.

Now I had the opportunity to talk with parents in their homes and to find out what had happened over the years. Many of these families lived in rural towns, straddling the border between Victoria and New South Wales. I'd met some of them years earlier, so this would be a chance to find out whether their lives had changed.

I first met Mrs Bannon three months after her son Doug had been diagnosed with a neurological impairment. The address on my list turned out to be a general store on the corner of the main street of a small rural town. I parked the car, and a dark haired pretty woman came out of the shop to meet me.

'I'm Marj Bannon and this is my friend Gina. She's going to look after the shop while we talk.'

The family lived above their rural corner store and had a nice

back garden at the rear. It was a lovely summer day and a table
had been set up next to the vegetable patch.

On my first visit, the pungent aroma of tomatoes drifted
around us as we sat at the table. Marj had plucked two red and
perfectly ripe tomatoes from the vine and arranged them on a
bed of fresh home-grown herbs. We sat drinking tea and eating
wedges of tomato on fresh basil leaves.

'These are delicious, the best tomatoes I've ever tasted.'

'Oh good, we have eaten quite a lot of them this week, so please
help yourself to more.'

Here was a young mother with a bubbly personality who loved
her garden, her family and everything else in life.

Marj talked about how she felt about Doug's disability and the
fears she had for his future. She also had a big worry about the
years that lay ahead.

'I'm worried about Doug's continuing dependence and how
this will affect my future life.'

I nodded but said nothing.

'It sounds a bit selfish but I'm worried about whether I will be
able to get around and do the things I used to do.'

'You are probably a very active person.'

'Yes I was usually on some community committee or other,
as well as managing our business and I really don't want that to
change.'

'Is there any way of organising things so that you can still do
those things?'

Marj looked doubtful:

'Doug is so active and gets out on to the road if I don't keep
an eye on him. His dad doesn't get home until after seven. I'm
worried that we might have to sell the shop. I don't want to do
that. I enjoy meeting the customers, particularly the regulars who
come in nearly every day.'

Marj talked about a whole lot of things that day, but we continually returned to the issue of how Doug's intellectual disability would affect her life. She called it 'The worrying issue of the month.' Marj was doing everything possible to make her son's life better but his diagnosis had challenged her expectations about her own future.

It would take some time to work through the shock of it all.

We parted good friends. I drove away wondering how she would be able to regain the life she wanted for herself, while continuing to take care of her son.

Five years passed before I returned to visit Marj and her family, but the shopfront address remained the same. We greeted one another warmly. It was a sunny day, so once again we sat in the garden. This time I had one of those wretched questionnaires for her to fill in. There was also another question I wanted to ask.

'I remember last time we spoke you were very worried about Doug's dependence. How is that working out now?'

'It's actually going much better. My husband fixed the fence and put a special latch on the gate. Doug is growing up and is easier to manage. When he comes home from school he plays out here in the garden while I work in the shop.'

'You told me that you had always been busy working on committees before Doug arrived, has anything changed there?'

'I suppose I've had to change. I'm on the committee at the school Doug attends. I organise fund-raising and you wouldn't find a busier person in this town than me.' Marj smiled. 'I need to be a busy person – that's just me. I represent parents on a local council committee and raise issues at council meetings.'

Marj had become a respected advocate for parents of children with a disability and somehow managed to continue to run her small business. It looked like she had found a new way to express her own identity and the changes fitted in with Doug.

I visited numerous parents and talked with them in their homes. Many had been devastated by the diagnosis.

When Delia was told that her son Dan would be intellectually disabled she was utterly shattered. She had done quite well at school herself and wanted her children also to do well and have the same opportunity to go to university and get a good job. She knew such a future was not going to be possible for her son.

I met up with her again as ten year old Dan came into the house from the school bus enthusiastically waving his latest painting. He smiled at his mother as though he already knew that she would like and be proud of his achievement.

'Oh look at that beautiful golden colour – just the same as our house.'

When the painting was flashed in front of me I caught sight of the shape of a house and a big splash of yellow paint. A teacher had written the title of the painting 'HOME'. Delia gave her son an affectionate hug as he went to hang his school bag in the hallway.

It looked as if Delia's disappointment about Dan not being able to go to university had been completely dispelled. Later, she confided that her older non-disabled son had decided not to go to university either. But Delia felt that the disappointment had been greater with Dan:

'It was just another difficult thing we had to deal with straight away after the diagnosis. The adjustment to my eldest son's education has been gradual and we had time to get used to it.'

Delia knew that life would always be challenging, but she believed that Dan's 'cheerful and affectionate personality' would be a sufficient reward. I thought that comforting family relationships would also help. I left them gathering kiwi fruit from the vine growing over the front deck and heard Delia say:

'Put the basket on the deck Dan.'

Dan took a basket from the table and placed it carefully under the vine.

'Here are some ripe ones for the basket.'

Dan took the fruit from his mother and put them in the basket before going back for some more.

'Take these over to Chris.'

Dan gave me two beautiful furry golden fruits through the window of the car.

'Thank you Dan, I'll eat them when I get back to the hotel.'

Dan gave me a wide open smile. Delia's face was beaming:

'Goodbye. See you again soon.'

The next day I drove west following the course of the river Murray. Mothers were usually more eager to talk with me than fathers. But Mr Daniel had been happy to volunteer. We talked a year after a road accident in which his wife had died and his son Ben was left neurologically impaired.

'I will never be able to forgive myself for what happened to my wife, and to Ben.'

Mr Daniel was struggling with his feelings about the accident. It turned out that he had been driving the family car. His son Ben had been described as a slow learner. He talked about his reactions with tears in his eyes and recalled his loneliness and worry about how Ben would develop. Uncertainty about the future was a big problem:

'I'm worried about whether he will be able to go to school and get a job or whether he will be dependent on me for the rest of his life.'

On my second visit Mr Daniel told me that he had been lucky to have the assistance of Ben's grandmother, and that his own problems, caused by the accident, had greatly improved:

'The year before last was a very difficult one because Ben's behaviour went into decline. But a teacher gave me some useful information about how to manage him and that made a big difference.'

'How has Ben developed since then?'

'A year ago he began to improve really quickly and regained some of the skills he had lost. Now he's attending the local primary school down the road.'

Support from a teacher and Ben's grandmother had made it possible for this father to cope. The family was flourishing.

Some of the families I visited lived on small farms away from rural towns. I never did fully master the technique for opening and then fastening big heavy farm gates while trying to keep my balance on the cattle grids that often straddled the road. Suitable farm shoes were always in the boot of the car.

When I parked the car under the wisteria-covered car port of a farm house in northern Victoria, I sighed with relief at having finally made it to the door. Under a clump of trees I could see Jan, who had all the features of Down syndrome, playing with her sister and two dogs in a very large garden. The children waved, the dogs barked and Jan's mother, wearing a voluminous country apron, welcomed me at the door. Later we sat drinking tea, eating freshly baked scones and chatting in the back garden. The diagnosis of Down syndrome had happened years earlier, soon after Jan was born. Her mum had been lucky to get into a parent group in one of the lager towns. Now she could talk to other mums. So what was her reaction to her daughter's diagnosis?

'At first I was shocked that Jan wouldn't be like my other children.'

Then she had started to think: 'She needs to be cared for just the same as the others. She needs to be loved like the others – even more so than the others really.'

Jan came over to sit on her mother's knee, and that's when her mum added:

'I just got on with bringing her up and now just look at her –
she's wonderful.'

And she was.

These were many good news stories about stressed parents
who had managed to get help from extended family and services
and were eventually able to cope. But for every such family, I
knew many others who couldn't get the help they needed.

There were some excellent programs for parents in every
state of Australia. But these were few and far between and too
many parents were on a waiting list that was far too long. Many
would never get to use the service at all. Some parents just gave
up.

The people I worked with in disability services were of the
same view: Parents, as well as their disabled family member,
should be able to have a reasonably normal life. Whenever I
talked with friends about these issues we always came back to
the same point of agreement: 'Parents shouldn't be so overly
burdened with caring for their child that siblings and their own
relationships suffer.'

Many families didn't have the services they needed; nor was
there much hope that they ever would.

The people who run services tend to believe that they know
what parents want, and that's what they set out to provide. But
parents often want something outside the scope of existing
services. And they want flexibility in choosing what is right for
them. When I was invited to run some group meetings with
parents of children attending special development schools, it was
an opportunity to find out what this particular group of parents
believed they needed most.

In one meeting I simply asked parents what they most wanted.
There was a collective laugh around the room and no shortage
of replies:

'If only there was somebody to talk to regularly about my son, I need to talk to someone when I need to … yes that would be a big help for me.'

Another echoed this same desire.

'Talking to other parents and people who can help with information is what I most need.'

Some simply wanted general information about any service that may be able to help them. Others wanted quite specific information, such as:

'What to expect of my child and what I can teach her to do.'

And:

'Information that is absolutely practical by showing me how to manage his behaviour at home. Practical help like somebody who can just take over while I do the shopping or the ordinary things mums do.'

A young mother pleaded: 'I just want to leave him with a baby-sitter I can trust while I do things like getting my hair cut.' Quite a few of the mums nodded their agreement.

Some parents wanted help in managing social situations away from home.

'People stare at him when he starts to talk and it becomes obvious that something is wrong – it makes me feel bad.'

'He looks different to other kids, so people can't take their eyes off him and it draws attention to us all – and that's stressful.'

'When he walks around on his toes everybody stares. So how do I explain to people about his problem?'

For some parents, managing their child's behaviour in public was the biggest problem of all.

'She behaves like a much younger child, and that attracts attention.'

'He draws attention as soon as he starts to talk in his unusual way.'

'Getting his hair cut is a nightmare and embarrassing; he screams and kicks his legs. People will be thinking "Oh how terrible, fancy taking a child like that out in public".'

'The worst times were when people blamed me for not being able to control his behaviour.'

'We sometimes feel like we are on exhibition.'

'Everybody notices that he's different when he acts up, and they stare.'

'She acts like a two year old having a tantrum and I can't pick her up bodily any longer now that she's so tall.'

Donna was distressed because her young son was so destructive and out of control. She sat on a chair trying to talk through tears.

'I don't know how to manage a child with a disability,' she said. 'What should I do?'

Donna was expressing the feelings of helplessness felt by so many of the parents I met. She had coped with her first child when he was a demanding baby and toddler without any problem. But, like many other parents, she lacked the same confidence when dealing with her child with a disability. And she wondered 'How long will this go on?'

'I just don't know what is appropriate in his case,' she said.

Fortunately a teacher was able to help Donna and things got better after that. She was later described by the teacher as a very confident mum.

Later, when looking at my notes from these meetings, I realised that an underlying desire behind some of these answers was the need for somebody to give these parents hope. At one of the meetings a mother said it for a lot of parents: 'I just want somebody to show me why things will not be as bad in the future as they are now.'

And many of the mothers nodded their heads.

How could these mothers have hope for the future unless they could be reassured that their needs would be met? Once again, time would tell that story.

Chapter 22

Maya

Perhaps first born children are always the centre of family attention, especially when, in a new generation there haven't been any babies around for a while. Maya delighted our family, long after that day at Snook Cottage as a baby.

Lyn is a physiotherapist, so her Maya baby diary is filled with the pleasure of her daughter's very first dates in rolling, crawling and walking. Husband Tony loves sport and he too was pleased about his daughter's physical cleverness. He wanted her to grow up to be outstanding in some form of sport or another and said he didn't really mind which one. Even as a toddler Maya was tall for her age. Some of us thought that basketball and swimming were definite possibilities. She loved moving around to music and often copied the movements of the dancer on her favourite DVD. That's when my sister Honor and I decided that she was destined to become an actress.

Nobody thought for a moment that anything could go wrong in this happy family plan.

Every child is born into a family culture in which some things are valued more than others. Maya was surrounded by family members who appreciated creativity rather than unchallenged conformity. One windy day when she yelled at the autumn leaves falling around her as we walked by the side of the river, her reaction was seen as amusingly different. Her liking for things she picked up off the ground, rather than shiny new toys, was viewed very positively by us all. 'What a clever little girl,' was the usual comment.

By her second birthday Maya was striding out quite confidently. She was not at all daunted by the groups of people standing around with glasses in their hands. She pushed right through them. Somebody asked:

'Does Maya have a sight problem?'

No, she was heading for a piece of cloth on a chair at the other side of the room. Her whole focus was on the cloth and she didn't seem to notice the people holding their glasses in the air, out of her way.

One day at my sister's home I noticed that Maya had become very interested in lights and switchboards. She seemed to prefer things like this to any of the more usual forms of play. This was surely unusual for a two year old child. Should we be worried about that? Or was she just a spirited child who was interested in things other than toys? Nobody, least of all me, really wanted to know the answer to these questions. We talked happily about how Maya's dad, as a three your old, had been more interested in the drainage system than any of the toys in the garden. We had a proud tradition in our family of unusual and more creative forms of play. But unwanted thoughts kept hovering at the back my mind.

It was a relief when Maya returned to dancing to music. At one of our family lunches she danced on her toes all around the room while looking at her reflection in the mirror.

'At long last, we might have a budding ballet dancer in our family,' somebody said.

We all laughed with the pleasure of that thought.

Later in the afternoon, her dad took Maya by the hand and led her over to the sofa. Soon he was reading the story of three little pigs. Maya sat quietly enjoying the story. At the end, she wanted it all over again. It was a reassuring sight: just like any other two and a half year old child. A few niggling doubts persisted, but who was going to raise these issues? And who would that help?

Suddenly, Maya's behaviour started going downhill fast. One weekend Lyn, now pregnant again, took her to see her aunt in another city. The plane trip turned into a nightmare. Maya had always been tall for her age so people expected her to behave like a child of that size. She screamed from the moment her mother tried to put her into her seatbelt. Then there was more screaming, because she wanted to get out into the aisle. A woman in the next seat turned to Lyn saying: 'Can't you control your child?'

And that moment of utter despair, Lyn admitted: 'No, I'm afraid I can't.'

It was a relief to get Maya home from that trip. Now something else was on her mother's mind: 'How will I be able to cope after the baby arrives?'

Maya's risky behaviour was hard to manage. She didn't seem to understand that people were trying to protect her. One day, when she was about three, Maya was in the garden while her dad was working on the roof of their house. Tony was shocked when he suddenly found his daughter beside him. She was standing at the top of the ladder, on the edge of the steep roof.

Climbing a ladder was bad enough, but climbing over the back fence and running out on to the road, was even more frightening. Not for Maya, but for the driver of a car who screeched to a halt when she ran across the road in front of him.

Now we were all very worried. This had an impact on what family members were able to do with Maya. Lyn's mum decided to stop taking Maya to the playground down the road.

'I can't bear the thought that she might take a suicide walk straight off the platform and into thin air,' she explained.

A pleasant Sunday afternoon at the seaside turned into a potential nightmare. Maya refused to hold anybody's hand and ran off heading for the water. She was caught in time, but the horrific vision of her being swept out to sea was a worry.

Many family activities now carried risks.

At a birthday party, Maya boldly climbed up the yellow and red structure in the playground with her usual speedy ascent. Then, looking down to the ground, she stretched out her arms in the air preparing to jump. Her pregnant mother scrambled up the ladder to rescue her daughter. Everybody else looked on in dismay.

How would this family survive with a new baby?

Then a new development occurred. Maya's favourite new thing to do was to pull out the fluff from the back of the speakers. She held it up in the air, between her thumb and index finger and looked at it intently. One day she took the fluff to crèche and held it between her fingers all day. None of the activities at crèche that day could separate Maya from that precious piece of fluff.

Maya's behaviour was unusual and difficult to cope with. We next had to wrestle with another big question: why wasn't Maya talking like other children do long before they turn four? Although a crisis was inevitable it still came as a shock.

The head carer at her daughter's crèche asked Lyn to meet her. She wondered what the meeting could be about.

'Take a seat Lyn.'

The reason for the meeting soon became clear; it was a recommendation:

'We think Maya should be assessed by a paediatrician,' said the carer.

'Why is that?' Lyn asked.

The reply revealed a very specific focus for concern

'We are worried about Maya's expressive and receptive language development.'

'Yes, OK,' admitted Lyn. 'Maya doesn't understand what we say to her and doesn't talk like other kids her age.'

All of the questions and worries about Maya's unusual behaviour surfaced. What had previously simply been seen as not wanting to listen and follow instructions and having 'her own language', was now being professionally described as a problem. The new baby was three weeks old when the day of the appointment with the paediatrician finally arrived. Maya ran up and down the corridor at the hospital. Lyn and Tony tried to cope with a crying baby as well as their daughter who refused to sit down. In the end, the paediatrician was not prepared to give them a definite diagnosis but suggested the problem maybe 'a specific language delay' or a 'chromosome abnormality.'

He referred them to a speech therapist and wanted a review in six months. If Maya had a problem, we all wanted to know what it was, and the cause. Six months seemed an awfully long time to wait.

Families often act to defend against unwanted events that threaten any one of them. So it was in our case. Given my experience with disabled children and stressed parents I should have been far better equipped to help. I should have known some of the answers. I should, at the very least, have had some inkling of what was best to do. Instead, I was deeply anxious and no help at all.

When teaching, I had often thought that parents were in a state of denial about their child's disability. Now I was learning that their positive thoughts showed that they still had some hope. It meant that their dreams for the future were still intact. I was continually grasping at clues, suggesting that Maya couldn't possibly have autism.

In Canberra I'd been quite familiar with the characteristics of autism drawn up by the pioneering work of Mildred Creek. I had taught several children with this condition. This knowledge gave me cause to worry about Maya's tendency to withdraw and be in a world of her own. But Maya didn't seem to have what I believed was another essential characteristic of autism. She didn't lack affection. She often climbed up on to her mother's lap to give her a kiss. She loved the robust tickling game that my sister Honor played with her. And Maya often spontaneously sat on my knee. If rejecting close contact and affection was a major characteristic of autism then Maya didn't fit the picture. No, Maya couldn't possibly have autism.

I was grasping at straws. Perhaps I, too, was in a state of denial.

On one thing we were all agreed. Maya's unusual behaviour and slowness to develop speech was a problem that needed to be explained. The appointment with the speech therapist was therefore something we looked forward to with a mixture of hope and fear.

Meanwhile, my visits to the new services took on a new significance.

Chapter 23

Parents needing help

Over the years, I had come to understand that three pressure points devastate many parents. The first was the diagnosis of disability in their child. Then came their need for something to be done; an intervention early in their child's life. Finally, they wanted answers to their troubling questions. Some parents avoided further crises such as illness, separation or divorce, but many didn't. And if that did happen, the consequences could be catastrophic for them and their child. Now it was time for me to find out what was happening in services to families.

Being told that their child has a disability is a crisis for many parents. I knew from my experience with doctors in Canberra that the way it is handled by the doctor can make a big difference to whether parents were able to cope. I'd listened to many parents complaining about not getting enough help and information from the doctor. Finding out what happens in a paediatric clinic was therefore something I definitely wanted to do, but there had been no opportunity to do so. Now, thanks to some leave from the university, I was going to spend several days each month in a diagnostic clinic.

The hospital was one of the largest in Melbourne and, although it had a car park to match, it was surprisingly hard to find anywhere to park. People were coming from every possible direction and heading for the main entrance. As it was too early in the morning for visitors, I assumed they must have an appointment at one of the many clinics.

The children's clinic was on the ground floor and easily reached along a corridor from the main entrance. I passed a waiting area and walked down another corridor that led to consulting rooms for up to four doctors. Colourful brochures were available. A friendly nurse welcomed the parents and sorted out any administrative problems. And then Dr Phil came out of one of the doors.

'Hi Chris, come through here.'

We talked for a while and then he suggested that I should feel free to go into any of the rooms. However, on my first day, I chose to stay with him.

The task of telling parents that their child has a disability must be one of the hardest jobs in the world. I noticed that Dr Phil had organised his office so that parents would be sitting on chairs as high as his own. He listened intently to what they had to say. His sensitivity ensured that he was not only respected, but also liked. And parents showed it in their relieved smiles and 'Thank you doctor' as they left his room.

In my early days of teaching, I'd heard many complaints from parents about insufficient information about services from the diagnosing doctor. Now, providing information was just a routine part of what these doctors did.

Many of the parents I met were attending the clinic for the first time. Most already knew that their child's behaviour was not the same as that of other children of the same age and most had suspected a problem before coming to the clinic. Parents had waited a long time for this appointment. And waiting lists would be part and parcel of their lives from now on.

'Well here we are at last,' I overheard a young father say to his wife who was holding on to their restless child.

His wife mumbled something like: 'At least we'll know whether or not he has autism after this.'

Diagnosing autism requires a checklist rather than tests in a lab. These children often came into the room without looking at anyone in it and all seemed to be in a world of their own. Three year old Steve came into the office holding on to his mother's hand. Soon he ventured away. He had noticed some paper clips on the doctor's desk and started to line them up from one end of the desk to the other. Then he turned around looking for the next thing to catch his eye. That's when he discovered a reflective plaque on the wall. He stood fingering his image for a very long time.

Some of the parents I met at the clinic had been waiting for months to hear the diagnosis. Mostly, they recognised that something might be 'wrong', and there was often relief when a name was attached to the problems they had described.

Whenever I spent a morning in this clinic I tried to be in the foyer to watch parents as they arrived and left to go home. Meeting them was a revelation. The link between diagnosis and crisis was not quite as clear as I'd thought. Many looked worried and anxious when they arrived, but left the clinic looking more relaxed. Mums and dads usually arrived together. Quite a few children came with their mother only. In some cases, the diagnosis gave them a reason for their child's difficult behaviour. Perhaps that was why it was so often accepted with relief.

I came away feeling pleased about what I'd seen but wondering where parents went from here.

'So what happens next?' asked a mother I met leaving the clinic.

She was holding on to a colourful leaflet and expected that the diagnosis would lead to the next service in line. Whether she got that service depended on her own further efforts, and the length of the waiting list.

Parents were asking 'Where do we get help?' And 'where does our child get an appropriate program?'

That's where early intervention comes in. But whether a child actually gets access to such a service is often a matter of chance: Is a program available? Where does the family live? If parents themselves need assistance, is the program designed to help them as parents, as well as their child? And, equally as important, is the child lucky enough to be born in a year when services are available to help?

Then came an exciting change in policy. Family-centred early intervention was introduced and implemented in Australia in the late 1980s and '90s and because of my work with families I became immersed in the new legislation and what it meant. Changes were happening right across the western world. Once again special leave meant that I could visit services in Canada and the USA. That is where I met up with Roselyn Darling in Johnstown, Pennsylvania, and where we decided to write a book about family-centred early intervention.

Changes in the USA and other countries such as Australia had made parents a central part of early intervention. The views and needs of parents had to be taken very seriously by service providers. Parents had always wanted to be consulted and now, at last, it was happening. I wanted to believe that this would help to stave off a crisis in some of the families I knew. But early intervention was in short supply and many families missed out. Too many families didn't even know that early intervention existed. The potential for a family crisis was still very real.

By the 1990s many questions were being asked about families. What happens in a crisis because of illness, financial pressures or divorce? Who helps families that have split, or because of illness need temporary residential care for their child? Even the best early interventions programs in the world could not always avert these disasters. The few existing services were insufficient to avoid a breakdown in some of the families I'd known.

Even back then in the '60s we had wondered whether adoption

could have avoided Josh and Kip being placed in residential care after their mother died. But most people were sceptical about finding people prepared to adopt or foster a child with disability. Now there was another exciting development. Adoption and foster care programs for children with an intellectual disability were introduced in Victoria and I was invited to evaluate them both. These services were being run by foster care and adoption agencies rather than specialised 'disability services'. They were the much touted alternatives to residential care in a crisis. But many people were sceptical about their likely success.

Foster care and adoption had always been intended to help young children and their families when, for whatever reason, they were unable to cope. These programs were set up as a solution when support services hadn't worked and a place for a child away from their family couldn't be avoided. A good example of this was when a parent had a very serious health breakdown, making it necessary to find temporary foster care. If parents died, the agency would be able to search for a family to adopt the child. Sometimes foster parents themselves might decide to adopt the child. What an amazing alternative to residential care this would be if it worked. And now I was going to find out whether it was working for children with disability or not.

One day, when leaving a foster care agency, something caught my attention in a particularly compelling way.

A foster mother was talking cheerfully to Bo, a child I knew to have a severe disability. I had met his mother a year earlier and knew she had been struggling to cope with her son after her husband left the family. Bo's mother also had a health problem that meant lifting him was practically impossible. That's why he needed somebody to assist with his care. One day I caught up with them in the car park. The foster carer had already looked after Bo for several months and the social worker was keen to keep the relationship between him, his mother and the foster carer strong. She had organised regular meetings between them all in the hope that this would help them.

I took in the scene from the car park. The foster mum had already spent an hour with Bo's mother in the agency. Now the carer was leaving with Bo in his pusher. And his mother was walking by his side. I walked across the car park towards my car and saw Bo's mother kissing her son before leaving.

'Bye! See you again soon.'

The foster mum and her foster child waved back to his mother. It looked like they were the best of friends.

This was a truly wonderful sight. Here was one family helping another family, and that relationship showed. Both of these women acted as though they knew one another well. Of course, there would always be the potential for conflict in these relationships. But in this case there was no conflict at all and Bo's mother was very grateful for the help she was getting. She saw it as a crisis that would eventually be resolved. Meantime, she and her son were getting help while they needed it.

Everybody wanted the foster care program to succeed, so we had to find out whether the methods used to recruit foster care-givers were working or not. There was also the difficult problem of how best to match children with care-givers. Most of the foster carers had children of their own and I wondered how they would manage to cope with another child in their home. I later met up with the foster carer and she explained:

'My other children had to learn quickly to give attention to someone other than themselves.'

Was that hard for them?

'Yes, sometimes, but it is a very valuable experience. My eldest daughter often helps with Bo's care and now thinks differently about a lot of things. She is much more aware that some people need a bit of help in life. I think that if you asked her she would tell you that it's been a good thing for her.'

The chances are that Bo had found companionship and an additional sense of belonging within a foster family. Later, I found out that Bo's mother was eventually able to take him back into her home. And the foster care-giver soon had another child to care for. This was the perfect outcome.

We all came to understand that there are many different kinds of parent and many kinds of children. And in foster care, matching the two was what made it work for them all. The biggest problem was finding enough foster carers. That problem could not be resolved until a lot more money was forthcoming for appropriate advertising, selection and training of care-givers. One social worker I know still hankers for adequate funding for that.

Chapter 24

A family crisis

Every parent I ever talked with about their child's disability had a story to tell about a crisis affecting their family. Now one was about to unfold in my own family.

Sometimes we thought Maya's speech was improving. Her singing went on for the length of a song. She often sounded as though she was having a conversation with somebody unseen by us. But she had her own language. When her mum heard her say 'bee I tink' while pointing to the bee design on the sofa cover, it seemed like a breakthrough. Lyn thought that her daughter was saying 'I think this is a bee', but then Maya went on to point to flowers and animals on the cover, as though they too were bees. So the words didn't match the image at all. Much repeated phrases such as 'where are you going?' were in her spoken repertoire, but nobody was showing any sign of going anywhere, so the meaning of the words didn't make sense. The doctor had referred Maya to a speech therapist, which meant her name was put on yet another waiting list.

I saw many wonderfully charming aspects of Maya's behaviour. She loved to act out songs and sequences from films. At the age of three her repetition of 'Oh dear!' with a very distressed look, was better acted than the real actress in her favourite film. Films were what she wanted to watch from morning to night. But why wasn't she talking like other preschoolers?

Lyn knew that her daughter was slow to talk. She wrote about why she was slow in her 'Maya diary':

*'I think it is really because you are so happy in your own little
world of song and dance, and your funny little games.'*

Maya's mum loved having a daughter with such an endearing
and unusual personality. But she was somewhat concerned about
her speech.

Our ever-changing views about Maya felt like a rollercoaster
ride.

Speech was definitely a major problem, so we were glad when
the appointment with the speech therapist finally arrived.

At the first appointment the therapist said that she wanted
to find out what Maya could do. She sat at a table talking to her
and asking her to do things with various items on the table. Lyn
wasn't surprised that her daughter was more interested in doing
her own thing.

Lyn left the clinic still wondering what the therapist had found
out and what her assessment would be. She vowed that at the next
appointment she would ask a few questions.

Exactly one week later, Lyn entered the speech clinic with
her daughter for the second time. She had resolved to get more
information this time round. The exercises continued and once
again the therapist's requests were ignored by Maya. This was
exactly what happened at home, but here her behaviour was being
assessed. And that changed everything. Lyn saw what Maya was
doing in a whole new light.

Lyn struggled to contain her emotions for what seemed like
a very long time, but in the end she asked the therapist a very
direct question:

'What do you believe Maya's problem is?'

The speech therapist's answer was just as direct:

'I believe Maya is autistic.'

'Autistic?'

There was the word that the paediatrician had mentioned as one possible diagnosis.

That evening Lyn decided to do her own research on the internet.

'I need to find out,' she said.

After the children had gone to bed, Lyn switched on the computer and typed in the word autistic. That led to a page on characteristics of this condition. Lyn was at first transfixed, and then shocked. Later she told me that reading the list of characteristics of autism on the internet was like reading a list of Maya's traits.

'It described my daughter exactly.'

She still hung on to a sliver of hope. There would be no formal diagnosis until a full psychological assessment was made.

Finally, just before Maya turned four years old, the day of a very important appointment arrived. It had the potential to be life transforming, and it was.

The diagnosis was confirmed by the psychologist and the paediatrician. There was no doubt Maya had moderate to severe autism.

Still Lyn hung on to hope. And it showed up in many of her questions:

'OK, if that's the problem what do we do about it?'

'How can it be fixed so that Maya can catch up?'

'What is the solution, what can we do to make it better?'

Nobody was answering these questions. Perhaps nobody could.

Nearly two years went by. Lyn felt exhausted by the strain of coping with Maya's behaviour. It looked as if she had finally lost all hope. To make matters worse she was still on the waiting list for respite care in the area they had temporarily moved to. There just wasn't enough to go round.

I was very worried about Lyn and Tony. How does a mother

cope with an unwanted diagnosis and shattered dreams for her daughter? How do parents resolve their problems without enough time together to talk it all out? And what does an aunt who is supposed to know about these things do to help? I had written many research articles about family stress and coping with disability, but these were real family experiences. And everything that happened was charged with emotion and fears about how the family would cope. Academic knowledge tends to distance researchers from families and it was no help at all right now.

Lyn was trying to cope with a lot of problems. Grandparents and aunts tried to help out. But family members and friends had their own pressures and Maya's unpredictable, overly active behaviour was hard to manage. Nobody felt that they could adequately cope.

Family pressures began to surface in various forms. Numerous questions were raised. Surely it's reasonable for an uncle to purchase an entertainment unit for his family without having to worry about a niece who might climb on to it and unintentionally wreck it. Issues like this meant that some people didn't want a visit from Maya and her parents. And when an aunt wanted to celebrate her important birthday without worrying about her niece with autism, who can blame her for not including Maya on the invitation list? My sister Honor resolved her own problems by removing the precious things that she didn't want Maya to touch. She hid them away. It took a while to make the house Maya-proof but the water features survived.

There was much family support and understanding, but there were also very difficult issues to resolve. Maya's behaviour strained relationships. A family member felt that they had a right to give invitations in whatever form suited them, and Maya was not on the list. And Maya's parents thought that their daughter had the right to family acceptance. Friends went this way and that. They had differing perspectives. Everybody was right, but it didn't resolve the problem.

Maya was in danger of being excluded. And I knew what that meant: it would reduce her opportunities to learn. It also meant that Maya's mum and dad had fewer opportunities to get the family support they needed. It might mean that they all had to stay at home.

Then a more threatening crisis happened. Some of Lyn's problems cut hard into her sense of self. One day she saw a program on TV in which a presenter was urging mothers to 'Make sure you look after yourself.'

Lyn stared at the woman on the screen in disbelief. Then came her cry for help.

'What do you mean? Do you have any idea what my life is like?'

I could see that Lyn was under a lot of strain.

'It feels like I've lost myself,' she told me.

Her fortieth birthday was coming up and churning thoughts emerged in a momentous decision:

'I'm going to visit my brother in Singapore for my birthday,' she announced.

Even in the best of times, Tony wasn't good at birthdays.

'You want to leave me to celebrate your birthday with your brother and sister–in–law?'

Lyn was at the end of her tether and there was no easy way to snatch some relief.

I knew that the divorce rate for parents with autism and other disabilities was soaring to new heights. That's why there were so many mothers coping alone. I wasn't confident that the relationship between Tony and Lyn would survive. Lyn was under enormous strain and nothing seemed to be going right. If Tony left, how would Lyn cope alone? If Lyn left, what would Tony do? If they parted, how would they manage to give their children the care they needed? Bob said 'Don't worry; those two will be all right.' But my own anxious thoughts persisted.

One Thursday morning I got a phone call from Lyn.

'Hi Chris, I'm going to be away for a week or so.'

Oh! Is everything all right?

'Yes, Tony will be looking after Maya with some help from my mum and I'm taking Kade with me to see my brother in Singapore.'

Lyn didn't seem to want to talk.

'I'm in a bit of a rush; you can get the details from Tony.'

'Have a good break, and please give me a call when you get back.'

I sat down on a chair and wept.

Later I started to think about the way Lyn had reacted when Maya was diagnosed with autism. I knew that it had been a massive blow.

'At the back of my mind I realised that something was wrong with Maya because I just couldn't get her to listen,' she said. 'Until then it had never occurred to me that anything could go wrong with my pregnancy or with my child. I found it really hard to tell people about the diagnosis, it feels like a piece of me died when we finally knew.'

She continued: 'Perhaps it sounds rather melodramatic, but there is a kind of heaviness in me that I have carried since that day. An extra burden, a lifelong responsibility and grief all combined. It wasn't the big things such as giving up on the idea that she would go to university and get a job. I grieved more about things like Maya might never be invited to a birthday party or have her own friends.'

'I'm sure she will have plenty of birthday parties with friends,' I said.

Lyn picked up her own train of thought.

'When we went home after hearing the bad news, it just seemed to change everything.'

'How did things change?'

'It was hard to reconcile my previous ideas about Maya with her autism. Everything that I had loved about her; all her endearing funny little ways, her dancing on tippy toes and singing, sitting where she could see her reflection in the mirror. These were no longer endearing traits of Maya. They were due to autism.

'It felt like everything I had loved about Maya had been shattered by her classification as autistic.'

Then in one very painful thought Lyn revealed the heart of her internal conflict.

'I felt that if Maya had behaved in these ways because of autism, what was there left to love?'

There, it had been said; and now she was struggling with tears.

She needed professional help and support. We simply shared the tears.

Lyn left with her son for Singapore. She had arranged for her mother to spend a couple of days helping and Tony reorganised his work schedule to be home in time to meet Maya from the school bus.

When I visited Maya and Tony after Lyn left they were sitting on the couch together watching television.

'Is everything all right?

'Yes, this is what we do every evening, Just Maya and me.'

I looked at Maya and her eyes met mine.

'Are you all right Maya?'

Maya ignored my question.

I was walking over to the kitchen when I heard a voice so clear that I couldn't believe that it came from her:

'Mummy come home soon?' she asked.

'Yes, mummy come home soon.'

It was the first time I had heard Maya speak words that exactly fitted the situation. Perhaps emotion had cut to the core. It should have been a breakthrough to celebrate, but it felt more like a call for help.

Tony seemed to be his normal easygoing self and Maya sat close to him on the couch. And that's how I left them when I went out of the door.

Many months later I asked Tony what his reaction was when told that Maya had autism. I had always regarded my nephew as a person capable of smiling in a salt mine. So I wasn't surprised when he said:

'It had no impact on me at all.'

Did the diagnosis have any meaning for Tony?

'The unknown future was a bit scary but I wanted to focus on the positive benefits of autism and celebrate the interesting life that lay before us,' he said. 'I didn't feel any loss, because I didn't have high expectations. I had never dreamt about the perfect family life so I had next to no loss to mourn. Well. I must admit to the occasional sporting dream for Maya, but it meant very little.'

And had things turned out as he'd hoped?

'I was probably a bit naive about how hard it would get. We've had some very hard times. We are having one right now. But I'm glad that I had a positive view right from the beginning and that has helped me to avoid getting too depressed.'

So what did Tony want for his daughter?

'Long before I found out that Maya had autism I wanted to encourage her simply to do her best. I just wanted to be there for her. And nothing changed because of the diagnosis. I was never going to push her to conform to the expectations of other people. I just wanted her to be the best and happiest Maya she could be.'

Lyn and Tony had very different reactions to Maya's diagnosis.

And that was probably just as well. They were each working through their feelings in their own way.

Lyn and her son spent two weeks in Singapore. On her birthday Lyn's brother and sister-in-law gave her a chocolate birthday cake. They sent her off for a massage and organised dinner. She had a wonderful day.

The return flight had been arranged. My anxiety settled a little.

Then Maya's hope that 'Mummy come home soon' happened. Lyn rang me the next day.

'Yes here I am, and very happy to be home.'

For Lyn, this was a turning point. She had snatched some respite time and didn't want to look back.

Chapter 25

A regular life

It was quite early one Saturday morning when I walked into my local baker's shop to select food for an important lunch. The aroma of freshly baked bread filled the air and I looked forward to eating a breakfast croissant on my way to the institute. The baker had prepared rounds of filled baguettes and there was some beautiful fresh fruit to go on our platters.

The times were changing rapidly as we headed to the year 2000, and technology was an important part of that change. Children had computers in schools and technology skills were required of people entering the workforce. In the late 1990s I was team leader of a project to develop software suitable for disabled computer users. We called ourselves the equity access research and development group at Deakin University. Many computer users with disability had already given us some useful information. Now we wanted to test some of these ideas. This meeting with about fifteen people with disability would last all day.

By 10 o'clock the room was crowded. The range of walking and other movement aids, as well as some very clever but a touch territorial guide dogs, added a lot of fun to the meeting. Everyone laughed when Sunny the guide dog refused to let me through to the table at which his visually impaired owner was sitting.

'And I thought these dogs were supposed to be gentle and agreeable.'

Sunny kept his head hovering close to his owner, until his owner pointed to a place where he should sit. Sunny's owner was definitely his master and Sunny wasn't going to move for anybody else.

Every member of the group had their own story to tell and they were keen to have their say.

Wendy was an energetic woman in her 30s with long dark hair and a face slightly impacted by an accident causing brain injury. After spending nearly two years in intensive rehabilitation she wanted to open documents on the internet that would help her to find and keep a job. She needed software to do it.

Several people in our group had limbs that didn't work for walking, but they would be able to use a computer with a few adjustments. Trevor was keen to use an attachment that could be operated through his mouth because no other muscle in his body worked quite as well as his tongue. Jenny was blind and had worked for several weeks without pay in order to convince an employer that she could manage incoming calls. She needed to use a computer. I learned very quickly that no matter what the disability, whether physical, sensory or intellectual, computers can help.

Some of the people in our group had already become friends. Alan, who lived in a rural town, was keen to overcome some of his sight problems by using a computer. Alan's newly found friend, Geoff, had no sight at all but knew exactly what his additional needs were.

'I want to make documents talk.'

Such technology was already becoming more widely accessible on many computers. Being able to hear, as well as adjust the size of text in e-mail messages and attachments, was useful to many people without an obvious disability.

The equity access group developed several software packages to help computer users with disability. The most important and satisfying outcome could be seen in what this software helped people to do. And that purpose was made clear to us by the people in this group:

'We want to be employable,' they said.

'We want to get a job.'

Most of the people we spoke to wanted to get an ordinary job in the community. What would help them achieve this? Like Jenny, most simply needed some technical help.

But even though technology would allow them to do the job well, attitudes remained a barrier. Most of the people I met during this project already had the skills required for the job they wanted to do. They also had everything needed to make them very good employees. The question was whether they could find an empathic employer willing to fix up their technology needs and respond to their desire for a job. Where was the help they needed to make it happen?

In some ways our project to develop accessible software in the nineties was ahead of its time. Soon every computer would be programmed with features available to users whether they had a disability or not. Soon businesses would be more aware of the needs of a diverse range of computer users. That would make it easier for people wanting a job and also for employers. Technology was changing the way we communicated with one another.

There were many other changes occurring at the same time. The shift from specialist disability services to regular community services continued to grow in Victoria and many other parts of the world. Social workers, therapists, psychologists, medical practitioners, lawyers, teachers and early childhood workers were all being expected to adapt to the diverse needs of their clients, including those with disability. Almost all people with disability were living in the community and the community was becoming a little more accommodating of their needs.

Things were also changing rapidly in the Institute of Disability Studies where I had been employed for more than 20 years. It was now a very long time since disability was a sufficient reason for segregation in education and other services. Social inclusion was now a major goal to be achieved. In some ways the institute had become out of step with changes in services and the different requirements of students. Our courses and staffing were gradually running down.

Despite this, some exciting things were starting to happen.

People in the university's business faculty had already shown a strong interest in the technology needs of disabled workers. They were our colleagues and equal partners in our technology project. Without their skills the project would have failed to meet the needs of people with disability.

Many other departments of universities and colleges were also using their knowledge and skills to solve disability problems. People in departments of architecture, engineering, building design and planning needed to find ways to assist people to live relatively independently at home.

Horticulture was taking into account the diverse needs of people in garden design and maintenance.

Researchers in medicine, science, psychology and sociology investigated a wide range of disability related questions.

And education, along with all other professional training areas of the university, now had a responsibility to include disability related material.

Any list of faculties and departments with some relevance to the needs of people with disability would likely cover the entire university handbook. Every one of them can help prevent disability becoming a barrier to a normal life.

At my local gym I talked with James, who uses a wheelchair. Out of the corner of my eye I saw him using the same three machines that a very fit and athletic looking guy in red shorts had used only a few minutes earlier. I use one of these machines myself when I'm feeling particularly energetic. All these machines are wheelchair accessible and most gym users, including the very fit man in red shorts, would be unlikely to have noticed their additional disability functions.

What had been required to achieve James's access to the gym? I'm sure that lawyers and town planners had an influence on the building design. Designers and manufacturers of gym equipment must also have been involved. Awareness of the diverse needs of people within any community was required by them all. And probably, most essential of all, James was welcomed by the gym manager who requires all his personal trainers to know how to assist everyone who signs up for a program.

Children with disability are now included in mainstream services such as crèche, kindergarten, education department schools, recreation clubs, sporting venues and workplaces. Many different professions are involved. Their parents have needs that stretch into many other areas as well. All the professions are involved. The challenge now is to coordinate it to make it all work for people with disability and their family.

Change is inevitable. And it was starting to happen in the institute.

By the year 2000 in Victoria there were signs that disability needs and issues were being accepted into mainstream education and professional services. There could not have been any better resolution. Many of my colleagues had already departed. I was saved from redundancy because of my faculty wide teaching. But my time in paid employment was drawing to a close.

Chapter 26

Family and disability

Ordinary families often have a plan for what is likely to happen in the future. They usually expect that their child will get a job after leaving school or university and that they will become independent and eventually leave home and have a family of their own. So how does Maya's dad see her life into the future?

'What worries you most about Maya?' I asked him,

His answer surprised me.

'At least a couple of times a week she sits in a chair and cries for no apparent reason. I feel so sorry for her. Why is she crying? Is she upset at what she is missing out on in life? Is she just balancing her day from all the excited highs?' I have no idea what she is thinking and she can't tell me why.'

If only his daughter didn't cry, things would be better for her dad. Even if she could explain why she cries it would help. Would Maya ever be able to explain to people what is going on in her mind? How does she cope with a fragmented world that she doesn't yet understand? And is that why she cries?

And how does her dad cope with these sad moments?

'I suspect that if I think too much about anything to do with Maya's contact with the world I will probably get stuck in the trap of wishing for a more ideal world, and that's not reality.'

So Tony looks at the positive things about his daughter.

'It's easy to focus on the good stuff with Maya. She smiles as much if not more than the average kid, and she loves to play and to sing and dance.'

How does he see his relationship with his daughter?

'It is far from perfect, but it is a great relationship and we have such good times. I worry a bit about the future. Now she is only eight years old but what about the teen years and what happens as we all get older? But we'll manage, for sure.'

How does Maya's dad see the future?

'Maya is who she is and I don't want her to be anyone else,' Tony replied. 'Autism is a big part of who she is and I'm fine with that. Sure the future will be hard and there are going to be many times when I feel sorry for her, but is it all bad? No, certainly not. The future will be interesting, that's for sure.'

Family talk about the future for Maya reflects our uncertainty:

- What will happen to her when she leaves school?
- Will she be able to get a job?
- Will she have her own friends and people she likes to hang out with?
- Will she ever belong to a club?
- As she moves into puberty what will happen, and how will that part of a girl's life be coped with?
- How much help is she going to need as an adult?
- Will she always be totally dependent on her parents or sibling and how will they cope with that?
- Will she ever go on a holiday without her mum and dad? And will Tony and Lyn ever have a holiday break without her?

These are big questions about the future. But for now, everything is going well.

It's Christmas Day! And that means a family gathering. This year it was at Lyn and Tony's home. In the lull between gifts being exchanged and the meal of the year I noticed that Maya was missing. Her dad said:

'You know where she'll be.'

'Yes, there are too many people around here for Maya's liking, so she has retreated upstairs.'

I climbed the stairs and saw that the door to her bedroom was closed. Maya knew how to put up a barrier when unable to cope with a crowd. There was no response to my knock. So I knocked again.

'It's Auntie Chris. I'd like to come in, OK?'

Rhythmic sounds of 'mmmmm dododo asoo soo' came from behind the door.

I opened the door but couldn't see Maya anywhere. I spoke out loud, to let her know what was happening.

'Perhaps Maya is hiding.'

There was a mound on the bed and I knew that she was buried deep beneath the doona. I sat on a chair next to the bed.

'Hello darling. We are going to have lunch. Do you want to come downstairs and join us?'

Not a sound from under the cover. I tried to make it into a game of 'Where's Maya?', thinking that I would pull back the covers to reveal her face on the stroke of three. But she knew this game and held on tight to the cover. By then I'd already been rewarded with several muffled giggles. Suddenly, Maya let go of the cover and revealed her smiling face.

I looked around the room. Her dad is a builder and had worked hard to build this extension for Maya. She has her own bathroom, pictures all around and her belongings in a cupboard. Her favourite thing is on the wall next to her bed. It's a mirror.

In a way, the mirror gave Maya a constant companion. When playing, she looked at her reflection as though checking that the image was still there. When she moved, the image in the mirror moved and so she could control whatever her companion did. When she danced, so did the reflection. The two of them could be seen dancing and singing together like two stage stars in a chorus line. They moved arms in synchronised movement, touching finger to finger, nose to nose, and elbow to elbow. Maya and her reflection looked like best friends.

'I'm going downstairs now Maya. Come down when you are ready darling.'

I walked downstairs to join the family sitting round the table in the garden. Soon Maya appeared at the window and took in the scene from above. Lyn managed to get her daughter to move as far as the staircase, where she sat for a while by herself. Later she appeared in the garden. Her mother knew Maya would eventually realise that the invasion of people into the garden was 'not so bad'. It would just take time. And here she is!

'Hi Maya; would you like some turkey?'

There was a hairy sensation on my arm. Maya stood by my side, bending to brush her mop of curly hair against me. We touched in a companionable way and that started a well-known game. I moved my arm to touch hers and she moved hers back to meet mine. She went over to swing several times in the hammock before returning to my side for the touching game. Later I walked over to sit on the sofa next to Maya, not close enough to invade her space. Through the window I could see that family members were chatting on the deck.

'That's Adam wearing a blue shirt.'

'Blue shirt,' said Maya looking directly at her Uncle Adam.

So the game continued. I was so very glad that Maya was now saying words that were meaningful. She spoke in a deliberate and stilted form, as though it was taking a deal of effort to make the words come out. But the words were the right ones for the occasion. Hooray! She was making progress in leaps and bounds.

Maya had eaten quite a lot of turkey but very little of anything else. Late in the afternoon she went to find her computer communicator. With a deliberate touch from her finger she pressed a button that would get the attention she wanted. Her mother was putting a plate of uneaten food in the fridge.

Maya pressed a button and the message was loud and clear from her computer communicator.

'I want pasta.'

'I'll put some pasta in water to cook for you,' Lyn said.

So while the rest of the family recovered from another bout of overeating, Maya filled up on pasta in the kitchen. She had made her need known through the computer and her smile showed that she was as happy as everybody else.

Lyn, without knowing anything about my previous relationship with Rosie, had made contact with her and the organisation she runs. Rosie had suggested a computer communicator might help Maya. The new technology was working well. I'm sure that one day Maya will be able to say 'please Mummy can I have pasta?' and eventually she will be able to make it for herself. In the meantime the computerised communicator provides some useful assistance.

By now it was getting late in the day. I went over to the sofa to sit next to Maya, but not too near. After a couple of minutes she shuffled over to sit close to me.

Maya smiled.

I smiled.

Not a word was said.

We had bonded like kindred spirits. The most essential part of human communication had happened. We had understood one another. We sat contented and happy, side by side, while the rest of the family talked in the garden.

It doesn't always take words to communicate.

Chapter 27

Family, community and inclusion

Without families, life as we know it couldn't happen. If families didn't care, governments of the world would have an impossibly large number of problems to resolve.

In every community and every family there are likely to be babies and young children who are dependent and also older people with additional needs. Any member of any family could develop a disability requiring extra care. That is why the community cannot so easily be divided into those who have a disability and those who don't.

When an older member of a family develops a disability, how do we respond? That is a test for any family, including my own.

When I took my father home after mum's death, he looked totally bewildered. My mother had been the organiser of the home they had shared for so long. Now dad had no idea how to use a bank, or cook a meal that required anything much more than toast. It took all of the energy of my two sisters and I to organise everything previously dealt with by our mother. We taught him how to withdraw cash from the bank by himself. His fridge was kept well stocked with food and casseroles were always in the deep freeze. In time, the father we thought may never manage by himself ended up living contentedly, with a bit of support from us. But in his last years, he needed more.

Around the time of dad's 90th birthday, we noticed that an old war injury meant that he was losing his ability to walk. From then on he was glad of regular help from the local council workers. When his asthma symptoms worsened the district nursing service helped him with medications and personal care. In many ways dad had become more disabled than many people who had been disabled from birth. I thought of Jimmy and David who were intellectually disabled and sharing a flat down the road. They, too, had casseroles of food in their deep freeze and somebody to help them for an hour or two each day. On one of those days they helped to make the food that went into those casseroles. Despite their intellectual disability, they were able to do just about everything else by themselves. If they did have a problem, there was a telephone button to call for help. With adequate ongoing support in the community, Jimmy and David, like my dad, would manage OK.

Most families cope as best they can. But in recent years I've been struggling with an uncomfortable reality. The stress in families that caused so many children to be institutionalised during my early years of teaching has not ceased to exist.

The sad truth about the campaign for change in services is that while much was achieved for children and adults with disability, many parents were left with a huge task of caring. In Victoria the report to the Premier had recommended increased services for parents. Since then, government services have barely kept pace with population growth. And privately run services for families are limited by insecure government funding that could easily be withdrawn.

The international normalisation movement during the 1980s and '90s often side-stepped the issue of how families would cope. In Victoria, parents were given much too little attention. The anticipated focus on families was often hard to find. Existing agencies struggled to spread their limited services around. Parents were often viewed as impediments to the progressive changes that were being made. Sometimes, they were even viewed as the enemy of the new programs being set up.

When the institutions and hospitals were closed down we all

heaved a sigh of relief. But parents didn't have the support they needed at home. Their capacity to cope was crucial to the success of the deinstitutionalisation campaign but a lot depended on parents caring for their child at home. Everybody knew that demand for institutional care had to be eliminated, but it was the already stressed families who were left to cope without adequate help.

It shouldn't really surprise us that families often break down from the strain. Quite apart from the everyday problems attached to caring and coping with negative social attitudes as well as difficult-to-manage behaviour, the impact on the lives of parents and siblings is huge. I'm thinking about the parents who can't have friends over or visit their friends and other family members. And those who have absolutely no hope of having a holiday away from home. I'm thinking about those families in which only one parent can work. It is so often the mother who is forced to abandon her job aspirations in order to care for a child at home. I also know of many fathers who cannot work the hours necessary to secure a more desirable job. Others hanker for a normal life at home. And what about the siblings whose schooling and time with friends may be affected by their responsibilities at home?

The care parents give often stretches far into the future. Then comes the most challenging of all questions: 'Who is going to care for our disabled family member when we are no longer able to do it?' For ageing parents, this is often the most urgent matter to resolve.

When I called Ethel at her Phillip Island home on a cold winter day in 2011 she laughed when she heard my voice.

'Oh Chris, sorry I took so long to answer the phone but I was in the bathroom trying to solve a plumbing crisis.'

Then her problem with Rowan, now aged over 50, came out:

'Rowan has stuffed soap into the pipe while having his shower and I can't get the water to flow.'

Ethel was now in her nineties. She had had a bad fall a few

months earlier and when I later saw her at a party she was getting around with the help of two crutches. She told me that the accident had hindered her project about the flora and ecology of Phillip Island as well as her community work. Rowan was relatively independent and spent weekdays at a community house with his friends. But he enjoyed visits to his mother's house on the island. Showering was no problem for Rowan, but on the day I spoke to Ethel he had become distracted by the wonderful plasticity of soap. That's why he had taken off chunks of it to stuff down a pipe in the bathroom. It was still quite early in the morning when I spoke to Ethel and the problem was being sorted out. As always, Rowan was lucky to have his mother. But a depressing thought came into my mind: what will happen to Rowan when the inevitable happens and Ethel dies?

Recently Ethel set up a support group for Rowan. They will advocate on his behalf when she is no longer able to do so. There are financial matters to be sorted out and legal issues to be worked through a frustratingly difficult bureaucratic system. The desire to set everything right for Rowan is sometimes exhausting for his 96 year old mother. But, as always, she fights on. Again I found myself asking: should parents have to fight so hard?

Whether old or young, parents need support if they are to enjoy a reasonably normal life. In Australia, an early intervention package is now helping young children and their parents. Respite is available to some. But older children and dependent adults need support too.

Two big and central problems remain. While there has been a lot of talk about inclusion, the support needed to make it happen is often hard to find. If people with disability are to be truly included in the community, they need assistance to gain access to what that community has to offer, and to achieve the life that is best for them. My experience tells me that people with disability have differing requirements for achieving what they aspire to, and so do their parents. Existing inflexible services don't necessarily offer the combination of help that is right for them.

The second big problem is that something has to be done about the shortage and insecurity of services, and the long waiting lists. As long as funding is driven by the ad hoc decisions of political parties, the needs of people with disability cannot be met in a sustainable way. Funding available at one time may disappear in a flash when the government changes and different ideas about appropriate services fall into place. It is a problem experienced around the world.

In 2010 in Australia the rallying call came once again: 'The revolution is not over yet!'

It is normal in any community for there to be people with disability. Disability can happen in any family and every community and in any country of the world. Therefore it is an issue for the community, state and nation as well as for people with disability and their parents.

In 2011 the most exciting development by far in Australia was the move to find better and more secure ways of funding disability support into the future.

So what is this solution, and where do we go from here?

Bob and I were sitting in a local café one morning, reading a newspaper after eating our regular Saturday morning breakfast. Bob pointed to a section of the newspaper we were sharing.

'This will make you happy,' he said.

A year earlier we had both signed a petition, distributed by an organisation, to lobby political parties to approve the National Disability Insurance Scheme (NDIS). We knew that the ad hoc political way of providing financial support to existing services wasn't working. The newspaper reported how it could happen.

I was energised by the news. A disability insurance scheme is exactly what is required. Funding will at last be secure. People with disability may at last get the support services they need. Maya and her parents, along with many other Australian families, now have a very good reason to hope.

We live in increasingly diverse communities. Disability is no longer considered as unusual as it once was. Many people with physical and sensory disability have been living and working in the community for a very long time. But social attitudes still remain a barrier to some of the things they want to do.

People with an intellectual disability can now be seen more frequently in shops, parks and on public transport. They participate in fun runs and many other community events. They eat frequently at my local popular cafe.

But there is still a long way to go before all people with an intellectual disability or severe autism have enough friends, volunteers, advocates and facilitators in the community to be fully accepted within it. When I last took Maya around the zoo she started to make strange high-pitched sounds. A few people turned around, some stared and pointed at us; a few people smiled. Maya pulled a protective sun hat deep down over her head. I fixed my eyes on the elephants. A woman in the crowd came over and whispered:

'I know what you are going through. My son has autism.'

Standing there near the elephant enclosure we gave one another a friendly hug that showed our connection. It said 'we understand what's going on here.'

Many communities are now more accepting of the diversity of people within them. Some children talk or communicate differently. They may look a bit different, or act unusually for their age. Families still struggle to have a normal life. But now, in every group, there is likely to be somebody who offers an empathic gesture of inclusion. And there will be others who display the sincere belief that 'We all belong in this community'. Yes, things are definitely improving for the better.

These photos show happily engaged children in 2012. The photos were made available for publication by Noah's Ark. This service is now Victoria's largest provider of early childhood intervention and inclusion support agency services, with more than twenty sites across Victoria. It supports more than 1200 families and in excess of 2000 child care services to ensure children receive the best opportunities for growth and development and are included, supported and accepted in the community.

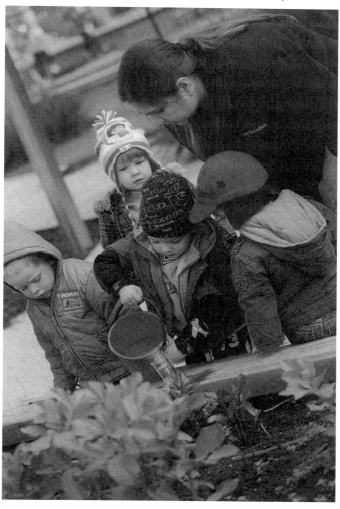

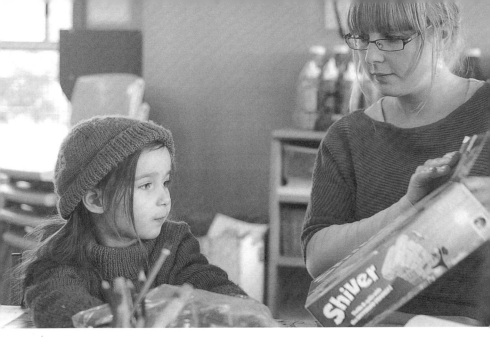

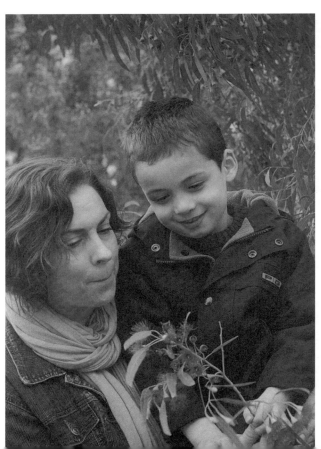

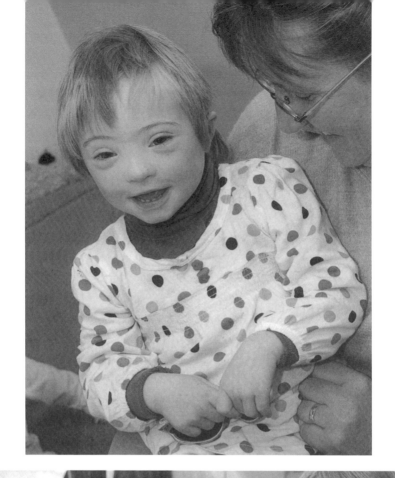

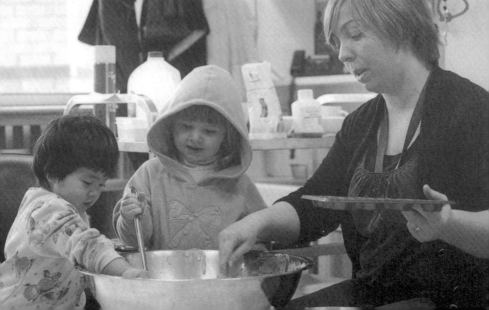

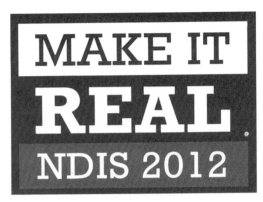

On 30 April 2012 rallies were held in every major city in Australia and in many regional towns. The national disability insurance scheme gives people with disability and their carers hope of a better life.

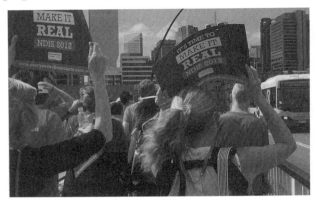

Image courtesy of cplqld.

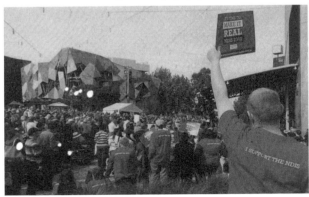

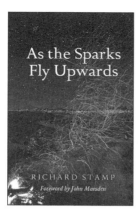
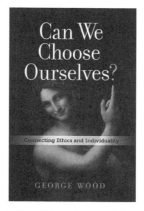
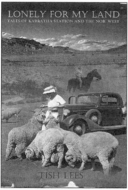
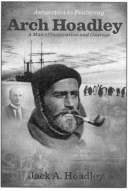
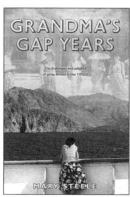
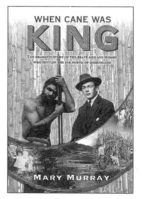

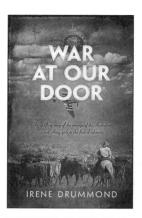
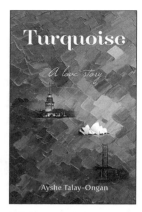
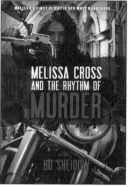
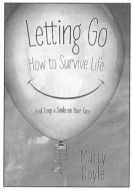
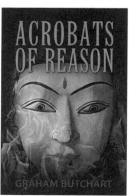
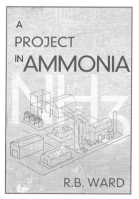